HOME FROM THE SEA

©1995 Mícheál Hurley

Main photograph on front cover
courtesy of
Walter Pfeiffer Studios
Dublin

Photograph of an 1825 lifeboat
from a painting courtesy of
Skegness Lifeboat

Photograph of 1995 lifeboat
courtesy of
RNLI Poole

Photograph on Back Cover
by Martin Walsh

Published 1995 by
Mícheál Hurley
Courtmacsherry
Bandon, Co. Cork
Ireland.

Hardback ISBN 0 9526007 5 7
Softback ISBN 0 9526007 0 6

Typesetting by Tony Moreau.

Printed and Bound by
ColourBooks Limited
Baldoyle Industrial Estate
Dublin 13, Ireland.

DEDICATED TO
THE COURTMACSHERRY CREW OF THE 1960s
WHOSE RUSH INTO ACTION UPON
HEARING THE BANG OF THE MAROONS
FIRED MY BOYHOOD IMAGINATION....
EVEN THOUGH THEY WOULDN'T LET US
SMALL BOYS INTO THE LIFEBOAT HOUSE !

Lifeboat Prayer

Merciful Father, all things in heaven and earth are held within your loving care, look with favour upon the Royal National Lifeboat Institution.

Protect and bless the crews of all their lifeboats and all who risk their own safety to bring help to others.

Guide all who work for the Institution that they maybe faithful to the vision of its founders, so that it may always be seen as a beacon of hope and light to those who find themselves in peril on the seas.

Through the same Jesus Christ, to whom with you and the Holy Spirit be honour and glory, now and for ever.

Amen.

CONTENTS

Author's Introduction		… …	x
Chapter 1	The Lusitania	… …	1
Chapter 2	Humble Beginnings (1825 – 1866)	… …	5
Chapter 3	A Fresh Start (1867 – 1879)	… …	9
Chapter 4	Overland Launch (1880 – 1889)	… …	16
Chapter 5	Changing Times (1890 – 1899)	… …	18
Chapter 6	Moving House (1900 – 1909)	… …	23
Chapter 7	The *F. S. Ciampa* (1910 – 1919)	… …	29
Chapter 8	The *Cardiff Hall* (1920 – 1929)	… …	31
Chapter 9	A Presidential Visit (1930 – 1939)	… …	35
Chapter 10	The Perils of War (1940 – 1949)	… …	46
Chapter 11	A Fond Farewell (1950 – 1959)	… …	48
Chapter 12	The End of the Line (1960 – 1969)	… …	54
Chapter 13	The Fastnet Race (1970 – 1979)	… …	62
Chapter 14	Crossing the Bar (1980 – 1989)	… …	70
Chapter 15	Towards 2000 (1990 – 1995)	… …	80
Chapter 16	For Those in Peril – A Brief History of the Royal National Lifeboat Institution	… …	85
Appendices		… …	91
General Index		… …	129

Part of the Coast of County Cork

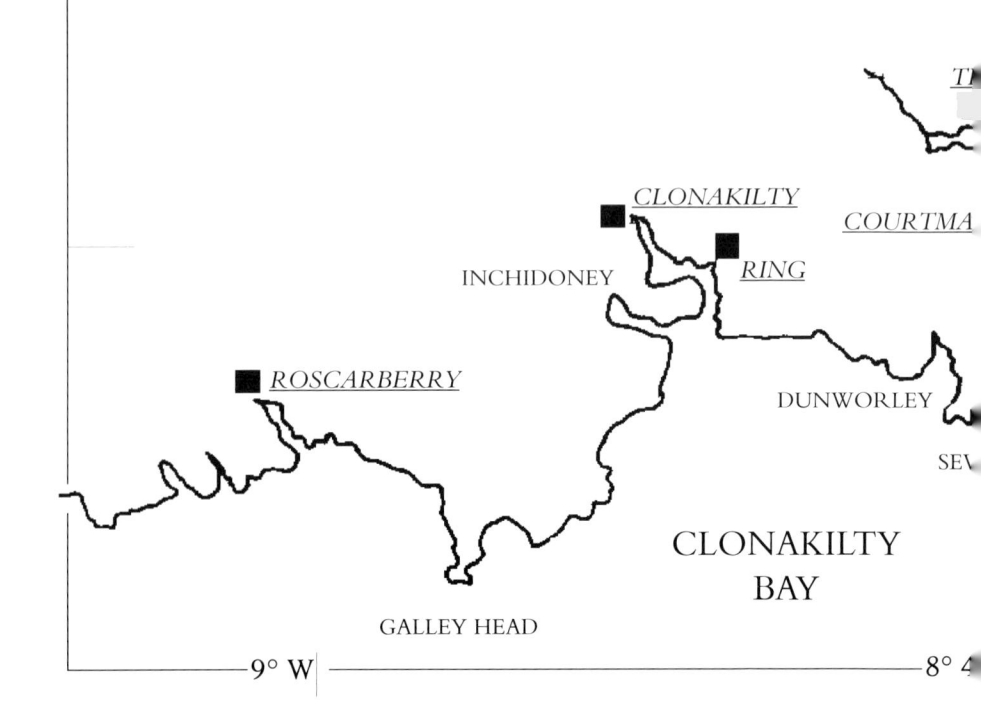

CLONAKILTY

COURTMA

INCHIDONEY

RING

ROSCARBERRY

DUNWORLEY

SE\

CLONAKILTY BAY

GALLEY HEAD

9° W — 8° 4

0 3 6
MILES

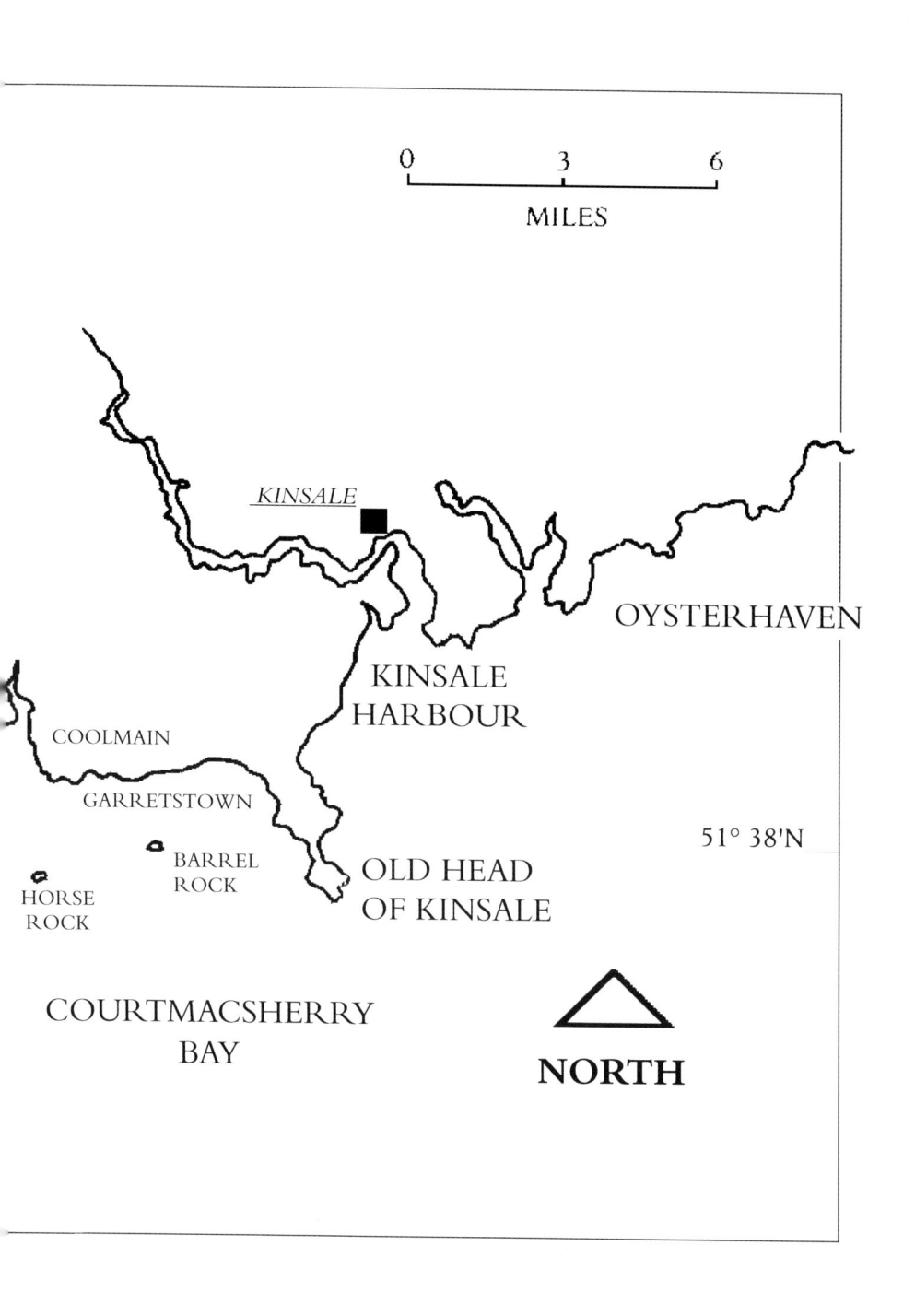

KINSALE

OYSTERHAVEN

KINSALE HARBOUR

COOLMAIN

GARRETSTOWN

BARREL ROCK

HORSE ROCK

OLD HEAD OF KINSALE

51° 38'N

COURTMACSHERRY BAY

NORTH

ACKNOWLEDGEMENTS

My thanks to all of the following for making this project a reality:-

RNLI Poole and Dublin

Desmond Bateman Hon. Secretary. Courtmacsherry Lifeboat

Jeff Morris Honorary Archivist Lifeboat Enthusiasts Society

The Cork Examiner for permission to reproduce so many of their Photographs

Donal Murphy of the Examiner Staff for his help in locating so many of the old negatives

Jonathan P Wigham Dublin

Thomas Mulcahy Courtmacsherry

P Lane H.M. Coastguard, Greenock, Scotland

Tim Cadogan Cork County Library

The National Library Dublin

Mr. Broughton Honorary Secretary Skegness Lifeboat

Llandudno Lifeboat

Exmouth Lifeboat

Dick Robinson, Ennis for encouragement and inspiration from his History of Valentia Lifeboat

Fr. Coombes Timoleague for useful history of the area from his book A History Of Timoleague And Barryroe

Michael Minihane Skibbereen

Barry Cox Honorary Librarian RNLI Poole

Barryroe Co Op for their sponsorship and the forebearance of their helpful office staff !

West Cork Bottling

Bernard Cronin and Liam O'Donoghue of Apple Computers Cork

Dave Mc Clelland, Barry O'Flynn, Brian O'Dwyer and Michael Cox for their kind patience with proof reading

Michelle O'Dwyer for all the typing in the face of some woeful hand-written scripts!

John Larkin & Paul Murphy for their assistance in getting a child of the '50's to make sense of the computer age!

Lastly and most especially my wife and children for putting up with the diversions from "normal" life in our house since last February.

HOME FROM THE SEA

CHORUS
Home, Home, Home from the sea.
Angels of mercy answer our plea, and carry us
Home, Home, Home from the sea,
Carry us safely home from the sea.

On a cold winter's night,
With the storm at it's height,
The lifeboat answered the call.
They pitched and they tossed,
'Til we thought they were lost,
As we watched from the harbour wall.
Tho' the night was pitch black,
There was no turning back,
For someone was waiting out there.
But each volunteer,
Had to live with his fear,
As they joined in a silent prayer.

CHORUS

As they battled their way
Past the mouth of the Bay,
It was blowing like never before.
As they gallantly fought,
Every one of them thought
Of loved ones back on the shore.
Then a flicker of light
And they knew they were right,
There she was on the crest of a wave,
She's an old fishing boat,
And she's barely afloat,
Please God there are souls we can save.

CHORUS

And back in the town ,
In a street that runs down
To the sea and the harbour wall,
They had gathered in pairs,
At the foot of the stairs,
To wait for the radio call.
And just before dawn,
When all hope was gone,
Came a hush and a faraway sound,
'Twas the Coxwain, he roared;
'All survivors on board,
Thank God and we're homeward bound.

CHORUS

I am grateful to Phil Coulter for his kind permission to use '*Home from the Sea*' as the title of my book
and also to reproduce the words here

AUTHOR'S INTRODUCTION

Most of us have romantic notions of the sea, how many of us have dreamt of sailing away from all our pressures with just the gentle breeze to carry us along. The sea, though, is a dangerous place and the coast of Ireland is littered with the wrecks of thousands of ships, many resulting in terrific loss of life.

The waters around Courtmacsherry are no exception, indeed as far back as 1656 a ship called the **Two Brothers** sailed for Jamaica, from Kinsale, and was driven ashore in Courtmacsherry Bay later that same day. Of the 244 officers, soldiers and women on board, 216 perished.

Shipping has always been busy off our coast either with ships heading up the Irish Sea for the U.K. or towards some local port. Since 1825 many of them have been glad of the services of Courtmacsherry Lifeboat. Though the nature of shipping has changed somewhat over the last 170 years the treacherous coastline remains the same.

In this brief history I will try to chart the progress of our local lifeboat which, except for a few brief breaks has remained at the ready for 170 years. I hope too to give a flavour of the community as it moved through so many generations and a few of the famous wrecks that are part of our folklore even though the lifeboat may not have been called upon to give assistance. It is almost incomprehensible that during it's illustrious career it has seen two World Wars, a War of Independence, a Civil War, the Great Famine and a Railway come and go.

There has been a common thread, though, linking all the decades and it is the very principle upon which Sir William Hillary founded the R.N.L.I. in 1824, that is, to assist anyone in peril on our coast regardless of race, colour or creed. Long may it continue.

I hope you enjoy reading my effort as much as I have enjoyed researching and writing it.

Mícheál Hurley,
Courtmacsherry,
September 1995.

CHAPTER 1
THE LUSITANIA

My grief on the sea ,
How the waves of it roll!
For they heave between me
And the love of my soul

Translated from Irish by Douglas Hyde

THE 7th May, 1915 at Barry's Point, about two miles South of Courtmacsherry village was a typical spring day. Mass emigration had not yet taken it's toll on this tightly knit community. At that time the forty or so small farmers and fishermen and their families who lived there were probably busy in the fields or fishing close by and the corn was growing nicely on the slopes of the headland that sweeps gracefully down to meet the waters of Courtmacsherry Bay.

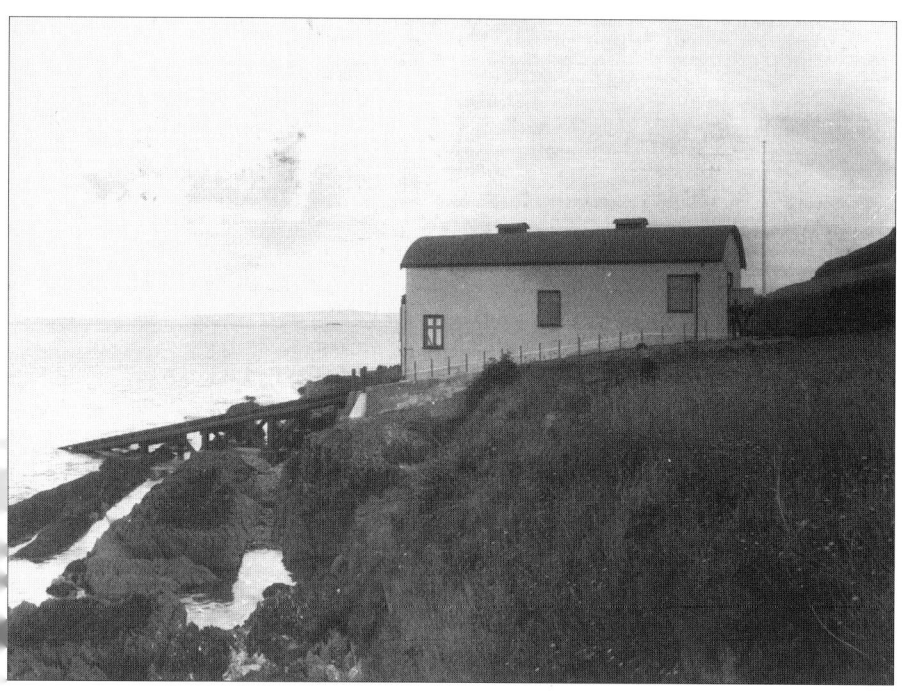

A rare photograph of the Boathouse at Barry's Point taken in the arly 1900's.

Photograph courtesy of Tom Mulcahy

Rev. Canon Forde, the Hon Secretary of Courtmacsherry Lifeboat, lived at Lislee House Presbytery, adjacent to the small church, about midway between Courtmacsherry and Barry's Point. The message that he got at 2.25pm on this flat calm sunny day must surely have stunned him. A large steamer was sinking about twelve miles off the Seven Heads and help was required. Heading for Barry's Point to summon Coxswain Timothy Keohane and his crew, he had no idea of the magnitude of the tragedy unfolding so close to our idyllic shores.

The men of Barry's Point were by now well used to the Lifeboat stationed among them since 1901. This would be their 10th service on the **Kezia Gwilt** but they could scarcely have imagined how their launch, that fine day, would be so vividly remembered long after the Lifeboat slipped gently into the narrow waters of Blind Strand.

On board with Coxswain Keohane at 3.00 in the afternoon as they set off were:-

Mike Keating	*John Murphy and his son, Jerry*
John Moloney	*Con Whelton and his son, also named Con*
John Moloney	*Paddy Crowley*
Mike Flynn	*David Moloney*
Pat Flynn	*John Keohane*
Pat Madden	*Lar Moloney*

Many of these were well used to the strain of the oar, either through fishing around the bay or on Lifeboat service.

In fact, most of them had been out all night in a howling gale, five years previously

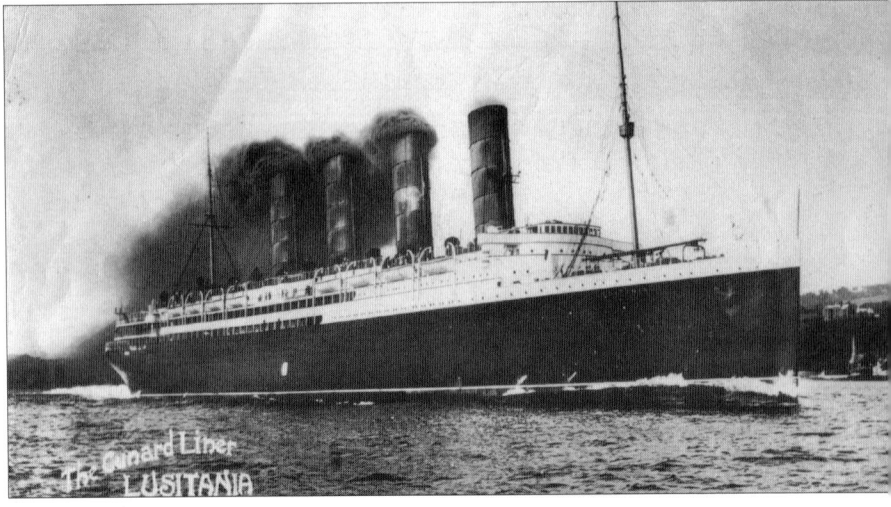

The majestic liner **Lusitania** courtesy of the Mariners Museum, Newport News Virginia

Photo kindly loaned by Paddy O Sulliva

to the wreck of the *F.S. Ciampa* off Dunworley. Unusually the Honorary Secretary, Rev. Forde, and Mr. Longfield of Seacourt House, in Butlerstown, a member of the R.N.L.I. Local Committee, also travelled out on the lifeboat. The drama of the day was witnessed by many people ashore, on the Old Head of Kinsale which forms the Eastern boundary of Courtmacsherry Bay, or on the Seven Heads only a mile or two South of the Lifeboathouse itself.

In Butlerstown, the school children were playing in the yard, grateful for the spring sunshine. As their attention was suddenly drawn by a loud bang out to sea, they were to be witnesses to the end of a great ship. The teacher asked the children to compose an essay on what they witnessed and they feverishly set about their task.

On the *Kezia Gwilt* too, no time was wasted as they pulled as hard as their bodies would allow, the fine day had ruled out the use of sails with which the lifeboat was equipped. On their way to the wreck, they met several ships lifeboats crammed with survivors. This was the first news they had that it was the famous *Lusitania* that had been torpedoed by a German submarine.

The *Lusitania* was the pride of the Cunard fleet, a ship of immense proportions, 785feet long, 88 feet wide and of 41,440 tons displacement. One of the fastest liners ever built the *Lusitania* was capable of a speed of 26 knots from her 68,000 horsepower turbine engines. On board were a total of 1,959 passengers who had left New York on May 1st. for Liverpool. Warnings had been issued in New York that U-Boats were active in the area and it was no idle threat.

On May 5th the *Earl of Latham* was sunk by the same submarine, again off the Old Head of Kinsale. The following day the *Candidate* and the *Centurion* were both sunk by U. 20 South of the Saltee Islands on the Wexford coast. Soon the majestic hull of the *Lusitania* would be in her sights.

At 2.10pm U.20, commanded by 30 year old Walter Schweiger, fired a single torpedo from a distance of 750 yards. Captain Turner, the Master of the Lusitania, saw the wake from the navigation bridge just before impact. An explosion took place immediately followed by a second more powerful one. The great liner immediately listed to starboard sinking rapidly at the bow with her giant propellers rising to the surface. It took only eighteen minutes for the *Lusitania* to sink, in that time people tried, in panic, to launch and board the lifeboats. The ones on the port side were too far inboard to be

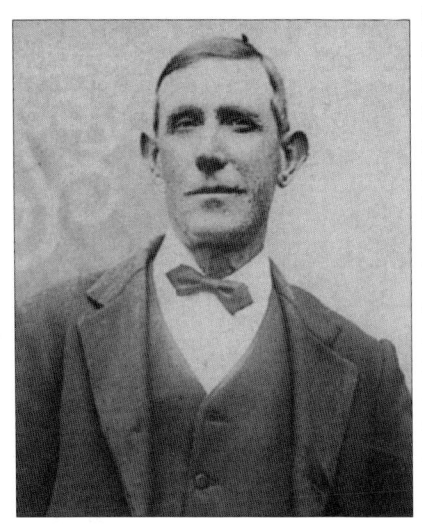

Coxswain of the *Kezia Gwilt*
Timothy Keohane
Photo courtesy of John Daly

easily launched and those on the starboard side hanging too far out to be boarded easily. Many passengers jumped or fell overboard from her steeply sloping decks. Only 764 people survived the disaster, many of the casualties were women and children.

Courtmacsherry Lifeboat arrived into this horrific sea of floating debris and dead bodies at around 6.00pm. The Queenstown Lifeboat *James Stephens No. 20* towed by a steam trawler arrived at the scene around the same time as the **Kezia Gwilt**. Both Lifeboats helped in the recovery and transfer of bodies to the warships and tugs that had arrived from Queenstown. The **Kezia Gwilt** remained at the scene until 8.40pm before setting out for home, they were towed part of the way by a steam trawler but still did not reach Barry's Point until 1.00am. The feelings of the crew and community are best illustrated by the words of Hon. Secretary, Rev. Forde, in his official report to R.N.L.I. Headquarters.

> *Everything that was possible to do was done by the crew to reach the wreck in time to save life but as we had no wind it took us a long time to pull the ten or twelve miles out from the boathouse which we had to go. If we had wind or any motor power our boat would have been amongst the first on the scene. It was a harrowing sight to witness, the sea was strewn with dead bodies floating about, some with lifebelts on, others holding on to pieces of rafts, all dead. I deeply regret it was not in our power to have been in time to save some.*

The selfless dedication on that fateful day epitomises the spirit of what the Lifeboat service is all about. Courtmacsherry Lifeboat has been back again to the site of the **Lusitania** sinking, on Sunday May 7th 1995, the Lifeboat crew laid a wreath over the wreck on the 80th. anniversary of the tragic sinking.

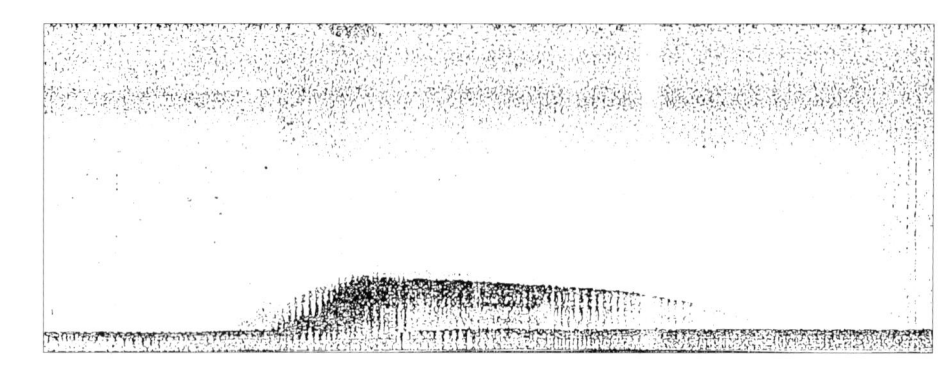

This is a record of the echo sounder on board Courtmacsherry Lifeboat on May 7th 1990, the 75th anniversary of the sinking.
It was obtained by moving slowly over the wreck from bow to stern.
It shows clearly the shape of the once great ship as she lies on the seabed.

CHAPTER 2
HUMBLE BEGINNINGS
1825-1866

Twas not without some reason, for the wind
Increased at night until it blew a gale;
And though 'twas not much to a naval mind ,
Some landsmen would have looked a little pale,
For sailors are in fact a different kind.
At sunset they begin to take in sail,
For the sky showed it would come on to blow
And carry away perhaps a mast or so.
From Don Juan by Lord Byron 1829--1824

COURTMACSHERRY at this time was only a small village. Smith's *History of Cork* published around 1750 described it as follows :

Lies under a hill, planted with trees that shelter it from the sea winds, and has a prospect of the harbour up to Timoleague. The coast for half a mile inwards from this place forms a semi-circle, where there are some good houses, and planted on a natural terrace above the water, which with Courtmacsherry, being encompassed with walls and turrets make a handsome appearance at a distance.

The terrace (near the tennis court) and Hamilton Row were built in the early 19th Century for use by visitors. The port was an important asset to the local economy since the transport of goods in or out of the area would be very difficult as the road network was poor. The coast road to Timoleague was only completed in 1823 and the road out to Butlerstown etc. was through the Earl of Shannon's estate (now the Hotel) and over narrow tracks. The Royal National Institution for the Preservation of Life from Shipwreck was, at this stage, in it's infancy having been founded only a year previously, in 1824. The name was not changed to the Royal National Lifeboat Institution (RNLI) until 1854.

To get an idea as to who was responsible for setting up a lifeboat at Courtmacsherry we must first look at the presence of the Coast Guards in the village. The introduction of very high excise duties in an Act of William III made smuggling a very lucrative trade which, in many locations, was professionally organised with special ships even being built for smuggling. The English government could not stand idly by and see a major source of taxation being taken from it, therefore, it established various organisations to counteract smuggling. One section patrolled at sea along the coast in cutters, indeed one was based around the Old Head of Kinsale to cover this area of coastline. In

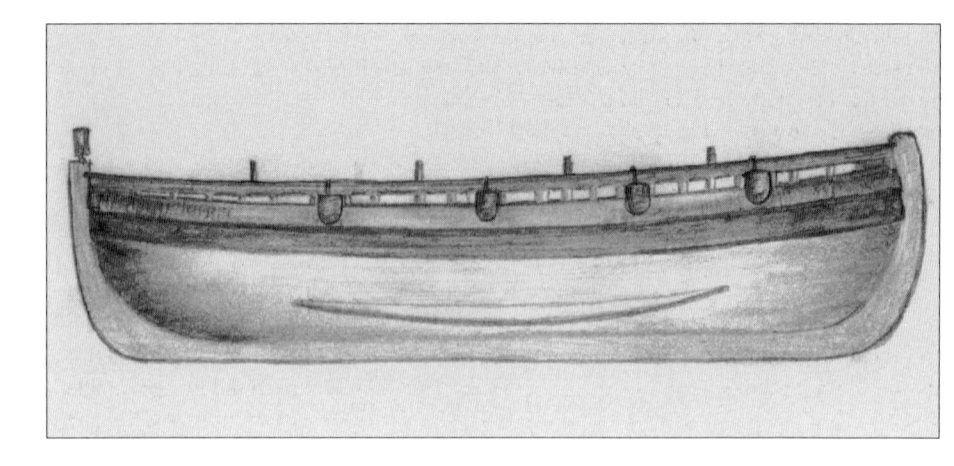

A sketch of the early Lifeboat, built by William Plenty
Sketch by Brian O'Dwyer

Courtmacsherry village the shore patrol was probably stationed in small rented cottages on the terrace in the centre of the village.

By 1825, the various arms of the Revenue Protection had been brought under one organisation which was then to be called the Coast Guard and it was achieving great success in the prevention of smuggling or in the movement on land of smuggled goods. The years up to 1825 had seen the Coast Guard taking on or being given many functions other than Revenue Protection. One of these, of course, was the rendering of any possible assistance to a vessel in distress on the section of coast within their care. This voluntary task was in 1829 to become one of the new list of regulations for Coast Guards then introduced. It is no surprise, therefore, that the Coast Guards opinion was sought as to the location of new Lifeboat stations that were being planned. Captain Dombrain, Inspector General of the Coast Guards, in Ireland, in July 1825, recommended to RNLI Committee of Management that the first choices for Lifeboats should be Arklow, Co. Wicklow and Courtmacsherry.

The Committee, in turn, asked him what type and size of Lifeboat he thought suitable and Captain Dombrain's recommendation was a 26 foot long boat. The Lifeboat which arrived in December of 1825 was built at a cost of £150 by a renowned boat builder, William Plenty of Newbury, Berkshire in England.

He had established a good reputation, as a builder of Lifeboats, and had supplied many to the Admiralty and the Coast Guard. Built of wood, the new boat was 26 feet long and 8 foot 6 inches wide, of extremely robust construction. It has often been described as a boat within a boat, the space between the two skins being used as large watertight cases giving great buoyancy. This new Lifeboat was purely a rowing boat and was fitted with ten oars. Part of the outer hull was also sheathed with cork to further assist the buoyancy and the boat had a curious feature of a gap below the gunwhale which apparently was to allow any excess water to roll out. It seems likely that the Lifeboat was launched by being pushed along skids to reach the water or transported to a launch site by whatever improvised transport was available.

Ironically the quality of William Plenty's design resulted in his not being asked to supply any further boats after 1829 as the boats were so well built the average coastal boat builder could not cope with repairs. There are no records of early launches and it seems that the Lifeboat was not protected from the elements by being housed. The Committee of Management received letters in 1829 complaining of inefficiency and, as a result, put the Lifeboat under the control of Lt. Rea, an officer of the Coastguards, who undertook to provide a crew at all times. For how many years more the first lifeboat remained on station is unclear but it, eventually, went into disrepair. Those in peril did not go unaided and on 21/2/1840 the sloop ***John and Ellen*** was wrecked en route from Newport to Courtmacsherry.

Lt. B.E. Quadling, the Chief Officer of the Coastguards, set out with seven other men in a local boat to rescue the four crew. The R.N.L.I. Silver Medal was awarded to Lt. Quadling for his efforts. Again in 1842, Lt. Quadling set off on February 7th with five

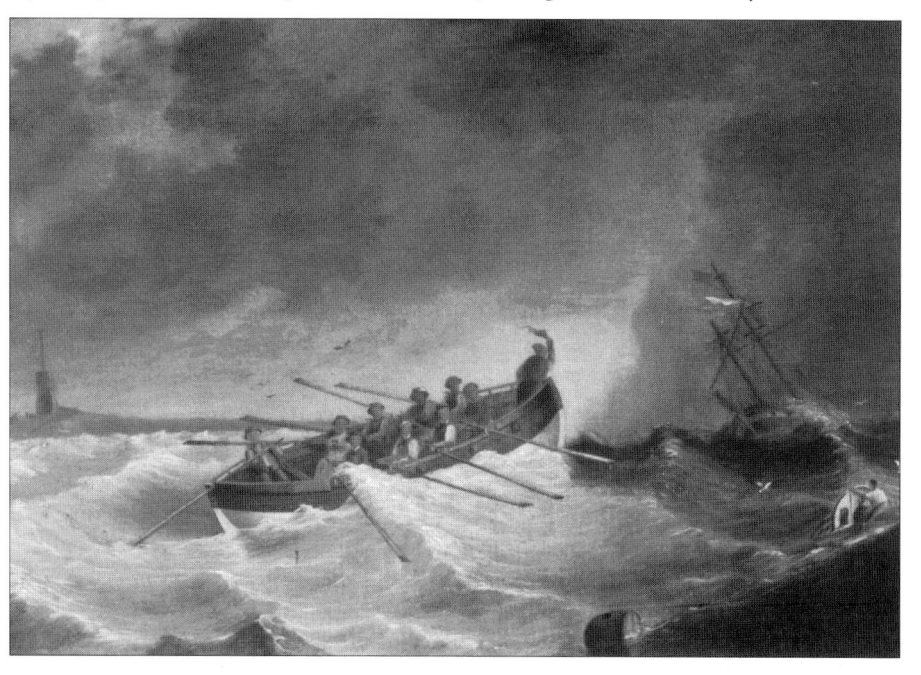

The only known painting of the early lifeboats as built by William Plenty This one is of Skegness lifeboat in Lincolnshire going to the aid of a vessel in distress.

other Coastguards in a shore boat to the assistance of the brig **Latona** which was wrecked at Courtmacsherry. They succeeded in rescuing the crew of 14. The R.N.L.I. Gold Medal was awarded to Lt. Quadling for this outstanding service.

By the 1840's the port was a thriving place and in one year alone 7,000 tons of coal were landed at Courtmacsherry pier from South Wales. Outward trade was equally busy with agricultural produce being shipped out to Cork and Dublin. Ten yawls were engaged in fishing and four lighters on the sand trade. Many boats were built locally as a boatyard was in operation on the site of the present tennis court. The dark years of the famine from 1845 – 1847, brought horrendous suffering to the locality and many new roads were constructed to provide work for starving men including the roadway from the 'church corner' to Lislevane. This roadway, to many, is today still known as the 'new line'.

Efforts to re-establish the Lifeboat were again made in 1858 when a new lifeboat was ordered. This craft was to be 28 feet long and 6 feet wide with only six oars. Built at a cost of £131, by Forrestt at Limehouse, London, she was considered too small for Courtmacsherry and thus not sent here. Instead she was allocated to Dover where she served until 1864. It was not until April 1866, however, following a visit to the locality, by the RNLI Assistant Inspector, that a new Lifeboat and carriage would soon be stationed in Courtmacsherry.

CHAPTER 3
A FRESH START
1866-79

> Who hath desired the Sea? — the sight of salt water unbounded–
> The heave and the halt and the hurl, and the crash
> of the comber wind-hounded?
>
> *From Songs of the Sea by Rudyard Kipling 1902.*

THE R.N.L.I. Inspector met with Captain Jones, an Inspector with the Coast Guards, and amongst their conclusions were that :

(a) a 32 foot long, ten-oared boat with carriage would be required.

(b) a local committee could be formed.

Captain Jones had agreed to take on the role of Hon. Secretary and would also act as Coxswain. This new arrangement would see the local organisation on a firm footing. A site at the end of the village was donated by the ladies Boyle and the tender of £171 5s by Mr. Edward Shannon for the construction of the boathouse was accepted. The boathouse had a large door at both gables for ease of launching and rehousing of the boat. The new Lifeboat was built for the sum of £249 by Woolfe at Shadwell in Norfolk and was funded by the City of Dublin Lifeboat Fund and was thus appropriately named ***City of Dublin.***

On Wednesday, February 7th, 1867, she was taken on her carriage in procession through the streets of Dublin and the naming ceremony took place at Custom

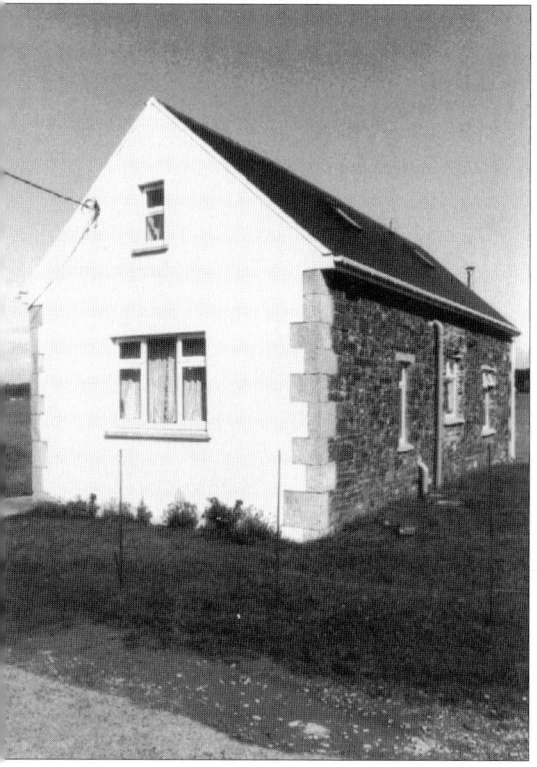

The 1866 Boathouse as it is today, the original building had large doors on both gables to allow the Lifeboat to be launched down the beach or taken to another location for launching.
Photo by Martin Walsh.

House Quay in the presence of the Lord Mayor of Dublin and many other dignitaries. The Lifeboat was then launched, off her carriage, into the dock with a crew then giving a demonstration of her capabilities. The Lord Lieutenant for Ireland in responding, eloquently, to a vote of thanks said:

> *it is difficult for us here to realise the contrast between these placid waters, this array of men and music, and the presence of these vast quays which bear the impress of giant human power and those scenes which the lifeboat we have just seen launched will have to encounter in its future struggles amidst the wind and waves - amidst the din of elemental discord and the cries of helpless human creatures, calling for aid and succour.*

The Lifeboat and her carriage were transported, free of charge, from Dublin to Bandon by the Great Southern and Western and Cork and Bandon Railway Companies.

On February 13th 1867, the **City of Dublin** was finally on service at Courtmacsherry where she was given a tumultuous welcome by a large crowd. The first service of the new Lifeboat did not take place until August 30th 1869, when she went to the assistance of the 140 ton Brigantine, **Wave of York** which had been run ashore having sprung a leak. The assistance of **City of Dublin** was not required as a fishing boat had taken the seven crew safely on board. In 1869 too, a new Coastguard Station was built on a hill

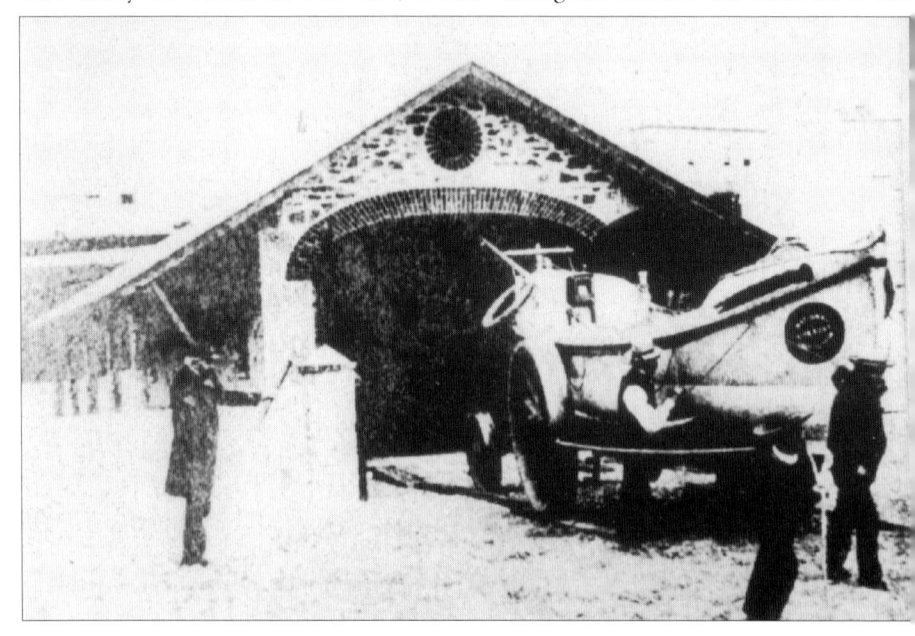

This is a photograph of the **Victoria**, Exmouth Lifeboat, Devon from 1867 until 1884. She was built to the same design as **The City of Dublin** but cost £5. more!

Photograph courtesy of Exmouth Lifeboat.

overlooking the village. One of the largest stations in Ireland, it was built by Murphy of Bantry at a cost of £3,270.

A relatively busy period for Courtmacsherry Lifeboat occurred in the next few years. Although the new boathouse in Courtmacsherry was less than four years old, it would seem that the Lifeboat Inspector wanted to try a new location. He had heard that the men of Travarra, a narrow cove, about four miles South of Courtmacsherry village, were great oarsmen and after some consideration it was decided to try the Lifeboat there for the winter of 1874-75.

A small cottage was rented for the winter to store the lifejackets and other equipment. During her brief stay at Travarra, the **City of Dublin** launched twice to vessels in distress. The first of these was on January 9th, 1875 in a South East gale to a large steamer, the **SS Abbotsford** of Liverpool, broken down half a mile to the West of Travarra. On the way to the scene the Lifeboat could see that the *Abbotsford* had been taken in tow by another ship, so the crew returned.

The busy nature of the coastline is evidenced by the varied destination of ships passing

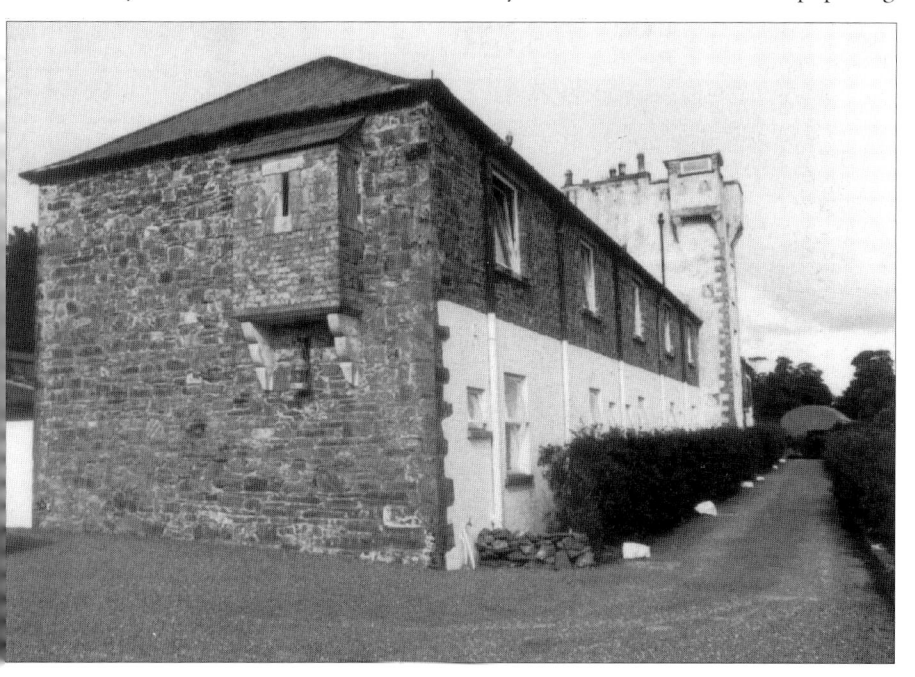

The Coastguard Station restored in 1970, was built in 1869 – 1871 at a cost of £3,270 by Murphy of Bantry. It was reputed to have been the largest fortified Coastguard Station in Ireland. A flagstaff was situated on the hill behind which was visible from the Old Head Of Kinsale. This was for Semaphore Signalling between the two places.

Photo by Martin Walsh

our coasts during these years. Another ship bound from Liverpool to the river Plate in Argentina with railway rails as cargo, got into difficulties on February 10th 1875. The *Hattie B* was a 250 ton barque with a crew of ten. **City of Dublin** Lifeboat left Travarra at 7.00 am and headed eastwards into Courtmacsherry Bay where the ship was anchored near Black Tom rock , a dangerous rock covered by shallow waters, about midway in the bay. The Lifeboat stood by for six hours in a heavy sea and ferried orders between the *Hattie B* and the steamer that arrived to take her in tow to Queenstown.

It is interesting to note that the crew at Travarra were completely different to those that normally manned the boat in Courtmacsherry village. Curiously, of the crew of thirteen on that day, three of them were Hurley in name. Maybe my cousins were involved in Lifeboat work way back then!

The Lifeboat's stay at Travarra, though, was short since it was decided that though the cove was very well protected from South West winds and the local men were an able and willing crew the road down to the cove was too steep, which would make it difficult to

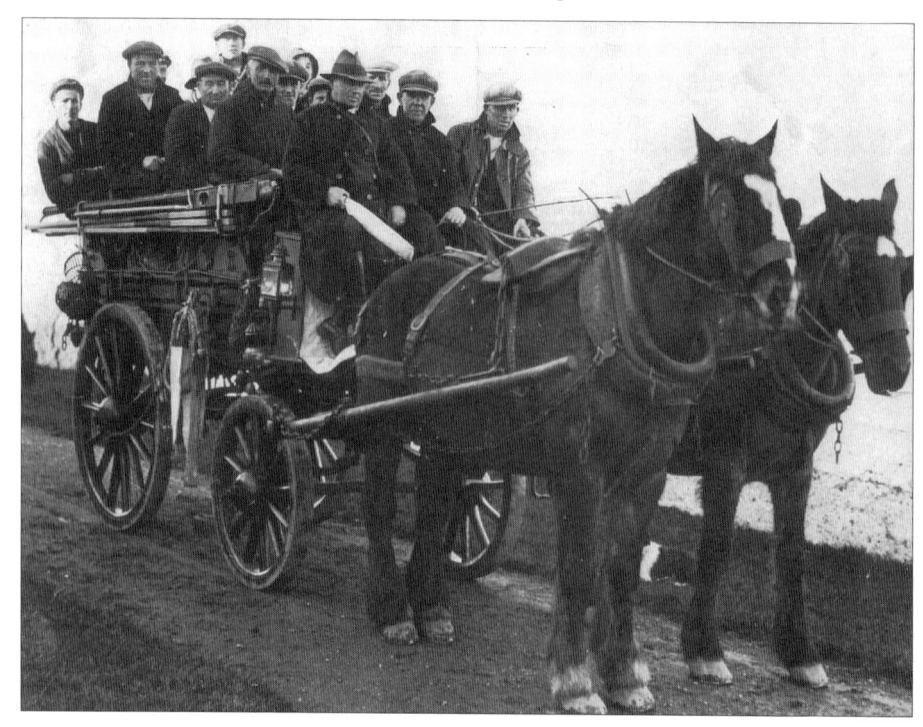

A fine example the "Rocket Cart" as it was known, this is the Guileen, East Cork team going to a rescue in 1924. The Courtmacsherry one was of a similar design and was housed in a small shed adjacent to the present Lifeboat house.

Photograph courtesy of the Cork Examiner.

haul the Lifeboat out of the cove to launch closer to a wreck around the coast. Another factor too was that the Lifeboat was originally placed in Courtmacsherry for protection within the Bay itself and not outside. Having considered all the factors, back to Courtmacsherry the *City of Dublin* came to continue her work.

December of 1876 brought her into service and showed the determination of Lifeboatmen to render assistance to a ship in distress.

On the 27th of that month the crew of thirteen tried to row out from Courtmacsherry around the Seven Heads and west to Barry's Cove where a schooner was anchored and flying a flag of distress. Having pulled for four hours in a South West gale and tremendous sea the Coxswain concluded he could not make it and so returned to harbour in order that the boat could be taken overland to Barry's Cove. Rev. T. McCarthy, the Parish Priest, of Barryroe parish was one of the local committee and having anticipated that the Lifeboat might not be able to make it, had six horses ready and waiting at the Lifeboat house. *City of Dublin* was placed back on the carriage immediately and headed for Barry's Cove.

Mr. Bunbury, the Hon. Secretary, went on ahead by horse and, on arrival at Barry's Cove, discovered that the ship had managed to sail away out of danger.

The Hon. Secretary rode back and met the Lifeboat along the way turning them back for home where the boat was eventually rehoused by 8.30pm.

The service had finally concluded nine hours after it begun.

Two further services occurred in January 1879. On the 12th, the 647 ton

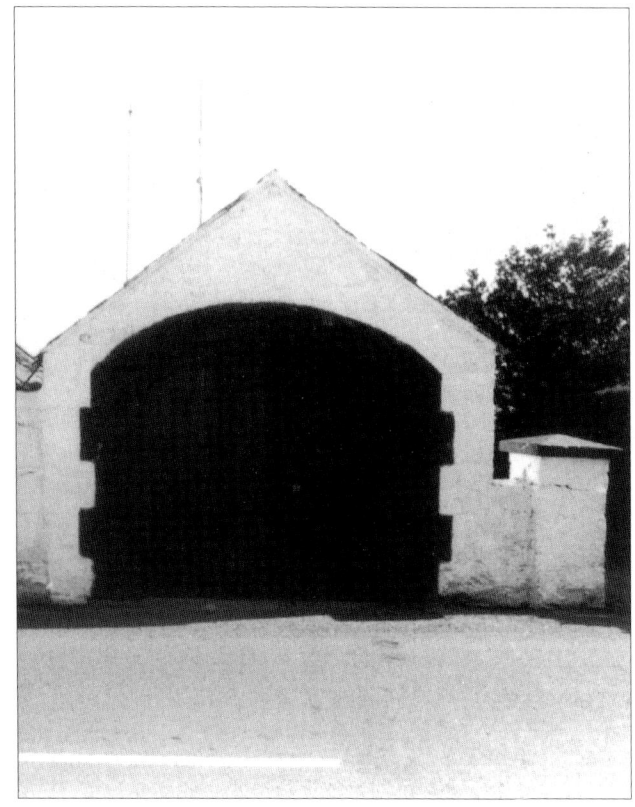

The shed used to store the Rocket Cart.
It is adjacent to the present Lifeboat house.
Photo by Martin Walsh

Barque **General Caulfield** of Newcastle, bound from New York to Dunkirk in France, with a cargo of wheat, had mistaken lights along the coast and grounded, on the bar, at the mouth of Courtmacsherry harbour.

There was a heavy sea due to the south westerly gale. The **City of Dublin** was quickly on the scene as also was a coastguard galley. The Lifeboat took off the eighteen crew in the afternoon, as the ship was by then quickly sinking, and landed them at Courtmacsherry. Ten days later another ship the **Nelson** was at anchor under the Seven Heads and in danger of being blown ashore in a south-east gale. The Lifeboat launched at 10.00am and the rocket cart based in the village, also left for the Seven Heads. The lifeboat was able to get a tow across the Bay from a steamer **The United States** which was looking for the **Nelson**.

One of the Lifeboat crew, Frank O'Driscoll, was a very lucky man, for when the tow rope from the United States to the Lifeboat parted, he fell overboard just managing to hold on to the Lifeboat's lifelines and hauling himself back on board. The **Nelson** was able to make her own way west when the wind changed to north-east during the morning. Slight confusion arose later on that night when people mistook locals gathering wheat

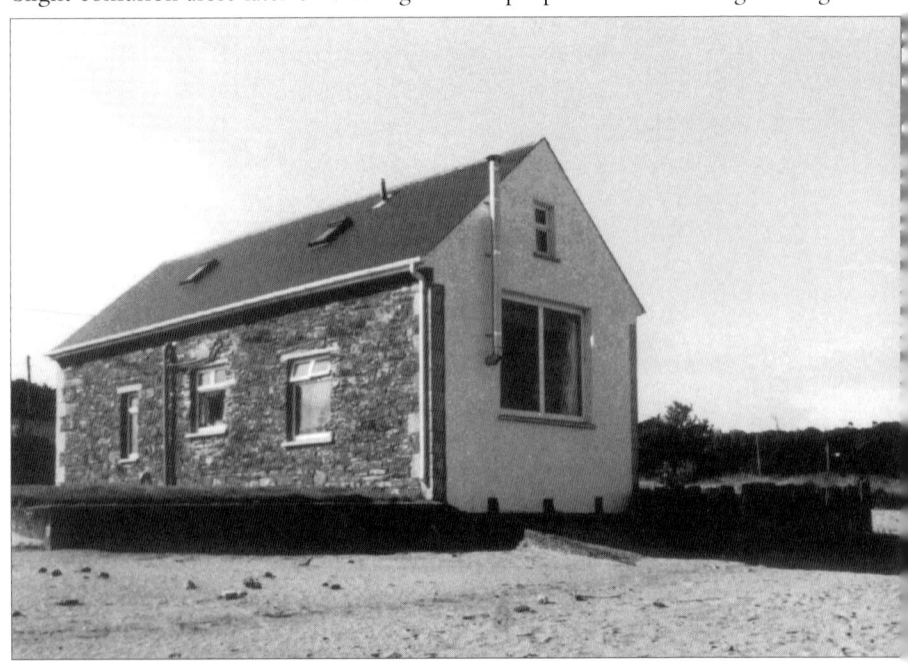

The old Lifeboathouse at the eastern end of Courtmacsherry village, which is now a holiday residence. This view is from the beach across which the **City of Dublin** or the **Farrant** launched so many times.

Photograph courtesy of Martin Walsh.

being washed ashore from the ***General Caulfield*** as another ship in trouble. Captain H. Townshend took over from Mr. Bunbury, who emigrated in 1877, a position he then held until the turn of the century.

CHAPTER 4
OVERLAND LAUNCH
1880 - 1889

The fair breeze blew, the white foam flew,
The furrow followed free;
From the Rime of the ancient Mariner by Samuel Taylor Coleridge

ANOTHER overland launch took place on 3rd March 1881 when a ferocious gale was blowing from the South East. A brig *Coleridge* of Newcastle was drifting ashore at the Seven Heads with a crew of eleven on board. The local committee decided that it would be impossible for the Lifeboat to get out over the bar without a tug so the boat set off on her carriage towed by four horses. While they were on their way south, a messenger arrived to say that miraculously the ship had got into a sheltered narrow cove and the Captain and crew had got ashore in their own longboat. The Lifeboat and crew returned back to Courtmacsherry to rehouse the *City of Dublin*. The *Coleridge* carrying a cargo of coal from Newcastle to Cork eventually broke up in the gale.

The last service of the *City of Dublin* Lifeboat occurred on 23rd January, 1884 when she was launched to assist a schooner which was in trouble at Broadstrand Bay. The *Hebe* registered in Cork, and carrying a cargo of coal to Bantry from Newport in Wales, was drifting having broken an anchor chain.

Curiously, this schooner was owned by the Murray family of Ring, (Clonakilty) and Courtmacsherry who operated several more as well including the *Thomas and Anne*, the *Catherine*, the *Mary Ann*, the *Thamar Queen* and the *Harry Herbert*. The Lifeboat ran out two more anchors for the vessel which arrested her drift and saved her. The *City of Dublin* since her arrival had launched 15 times and saved 18 lives. She had an ignominious fate being broken up a year later.

The replacement Lifeboat, which arrived in 1885, was at 34 feet, 2 feet longer than her predecessor. Built by Woolfe at Shadwell in Norfolk, at a cost of £300, she was named the *Farrant* since it was the legacy of a Mr. R. A. M. Farrant of Bayswater, London that funded the cost. Woolfe had considerable experience of lifeboat construction, having built sixty four boats of this class alone.

This new one carried ten oars and had a fixed rudder. She was self righting in design and had a launching carriage. Her official number(O.N.) was 103, but in fact, the numbering system was only introduced in 1887 by Mr. G. L. Watson on his appointment as Consulting Naval Architect to the R.N.L.I. All the Lifeboats already in service were retrospectively numbered.

The *Farrant* and her crew had a year to wait for her first call which took place on May 17th 1886 when she launched to escort a local fishing smack into harbour after she got into difficulties on the Bar. The crew, the Hon. Secretary recorded:- *"like the new boat very much"*.

Although it appears that due to the weight of the ***Farrant***, at three tons, being heavier than her predecessor, extra shore help had to be engaged to haul her up on her return from service.

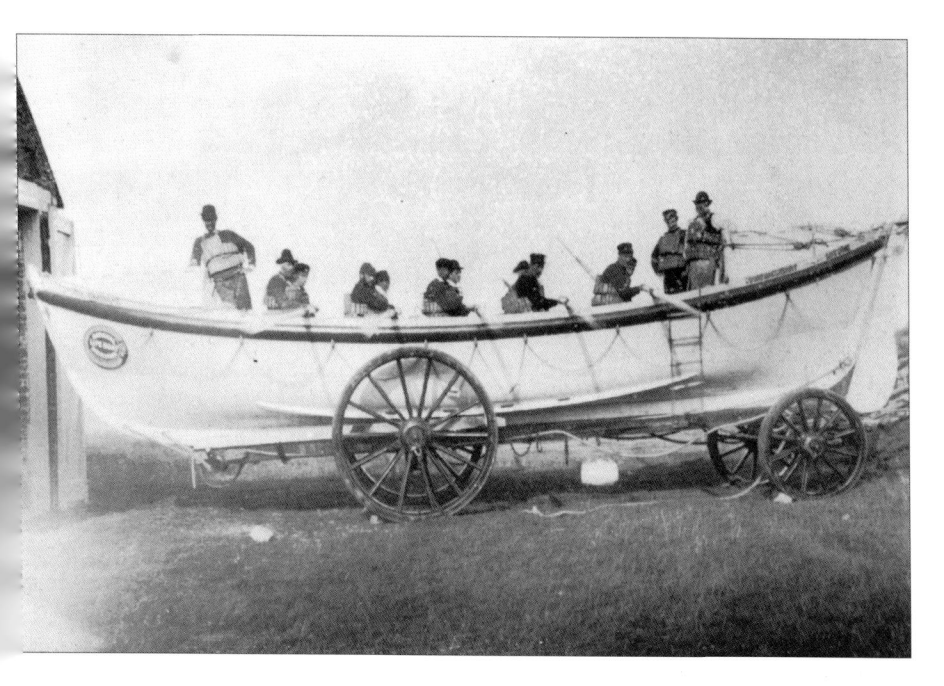

The ***Farrant*** Lifeboat, (O.N. 103) stationed at Courtmacsherry

CHAPTER 5
CHANGING TIMES
1890 - 1899

We left behind the painted buoy
That tosses at the harbour mouth ;
And madly danced our hearts with joy,
As fast we fleeted for the South:
How fresh was every sight and sound
On open main or winding shore!
We knew the merry World was round,
And we might sail for evermore.

From the Voyage by Alfred , Lord Tennyson 1864.

BY THE 1890's rural Ireland was being opened up more and more by the spreading of the Railway network. Courtmacsherry finally saw its first train roll in on the 24th of April 1891 and for the next seventy years it provided a major economic lifeline to the area. At sea, changes were taking place too, steam had now provided ships with independence over wind power. There existed for many years an overlap of technologies with sailing ships remaining well into this century. The R.N.L.I. was experimenting with steam to propel Lifeboats and in 1887 had ordered one to be built. For the men of Courtmacsherry though the power of the oar was still the only one they knew. It was to be truly tested in the early morning of November 13th 1891. The **Farrant** was launched to go to the aid of a large ship the **Gylfe** which was on the rocks at the Old Head of Kinsale.

The drama had begun at 7.00pm the previous evening when an uncertain report arrived to say that the lights of a large ship were seen near the Old Head of Kinsale. However, it was not until 1.00 am that a horse messenger arrived from the Coast Guard Station at the Old Head, to say that a vessel was in distress.

The **Farrant**, launched at 2.00 am with a crew of thirteen under the command of Noble Ruddock, the Coxswain. A southerly gale was blowing and conditions at the mouth of the harbour were some of the worst he had ever seen. After two hours of hard pulling the Lifeboat reached the Old Head only to find that the **Gylfe** had gone to pieces on the headland. Of the thirteen crew on the **Gylfe** only five were saved by getting up on the rocks at the Old Head of Kinsale through the assistance of shore help. Of the lifeboat crew that night, seven men were local Coast Guards. The Honorary Secretary Mr. Townshend, in his report, remarked that the lack of a telegraph station in Courtmacsherry had resulted in undue delay in getting word to the Lifeboat as the Old Head Coast Guard station was fourteen miles away by horseback.

The following year a spectacular wreck took place in Courtmacsherry Bay. On Friday evening July 1st 1892, the 3,364 ton liner, **City of Chicago** struck the west side of the Old Head of Kinsale. Commanded by Captain Redfern, she was owned by the Inman and International Line and was built by C. O'Connell of Glasgow in 1883. The **City of Chicago** had left New York on the previous Wednesday week bound for Liverpool *via* Queenstown. The journey was uneventful and having passed the Fastnet earlier in the evening just a short run remained to Queenstown. Thick fog had, by now, descended and lookouts were posted forward and speed reduced.

Then around 8.00pm the seaman posted forward shouted "*breakers ahead*" and almost immediately the fine ship went crashing onto the ledge of rock half a mile West of the Old Head of Kinsale lighthouse. The entire ship trembled from stem to stern with the impact and a certain amount of panic broke out among the passengers. The officers and crew set about calming the passengers' fears and distress rockets were fired.

On board the **City of Chicago** were a total of 360 passengers including some members of the American Peace Delegation who were coming to Ireland to observe the forthcoming elections. Amongst the 4,000 ton cargo carried on the liner were twenty bags of mail for Queenstown, 583 boxes of cheese, 325 barrels of oil, 92 bundles of rubber and a wide variety of other goods.

Upon seeing the distress rockets and hearing the blowing of the ship's whistle, the coastguards from the station at the Old Head were soon on the scene, as well as many locals. A rocket was fired from the shore and eventually a rope ladder was rigged from the top of the two hundred foot cliff down to the ship. All through the night, up this precarious ladder, around two hundred passengers had to climb and local carts took them onwards to Kinsale. Amusingly, one passenger remarked, after visiting the scene again, the following morning that if they had been able to see the height they were about to climb they might have preferred to stay on the ship but, with the thickness of the fog, only one rung at a time was visible. One of the Coastguards, Mr. Attridge, made over thirty trips down the rope ladder to help up the passengers. A small child had a lucky escape when, about thirty feet up the ladder, it slipped and fell. Another one of the Coastguards had the drama under control and caught the child before it could fall onto the jagged rocks beneath.

The rest of the passengers went around the Old Head to Kinsale by the ship's lifeboats and by the tender **Ireland** that had travelled out from Queenstown to meet the liner. The bow of the **City of Chicago** was firmly wedged in a crevice in the rocks and the Master of the liner had kept her engines running ahead all night to prevent her slipping back into deeper water. Salvage tugs arrived on the scene in the following day but a gale blew up and the **City of Chicago** became a total loss initially breaking in two amidships and eventually sinking to her watery grave. The **City of Chicago** has provided a rich pasture for divers over the years and the location is today nicknamed Chicago Point.

On Wednesday, August 3rd, 1898, the **Farrant** was launched to go to the aid of a ship

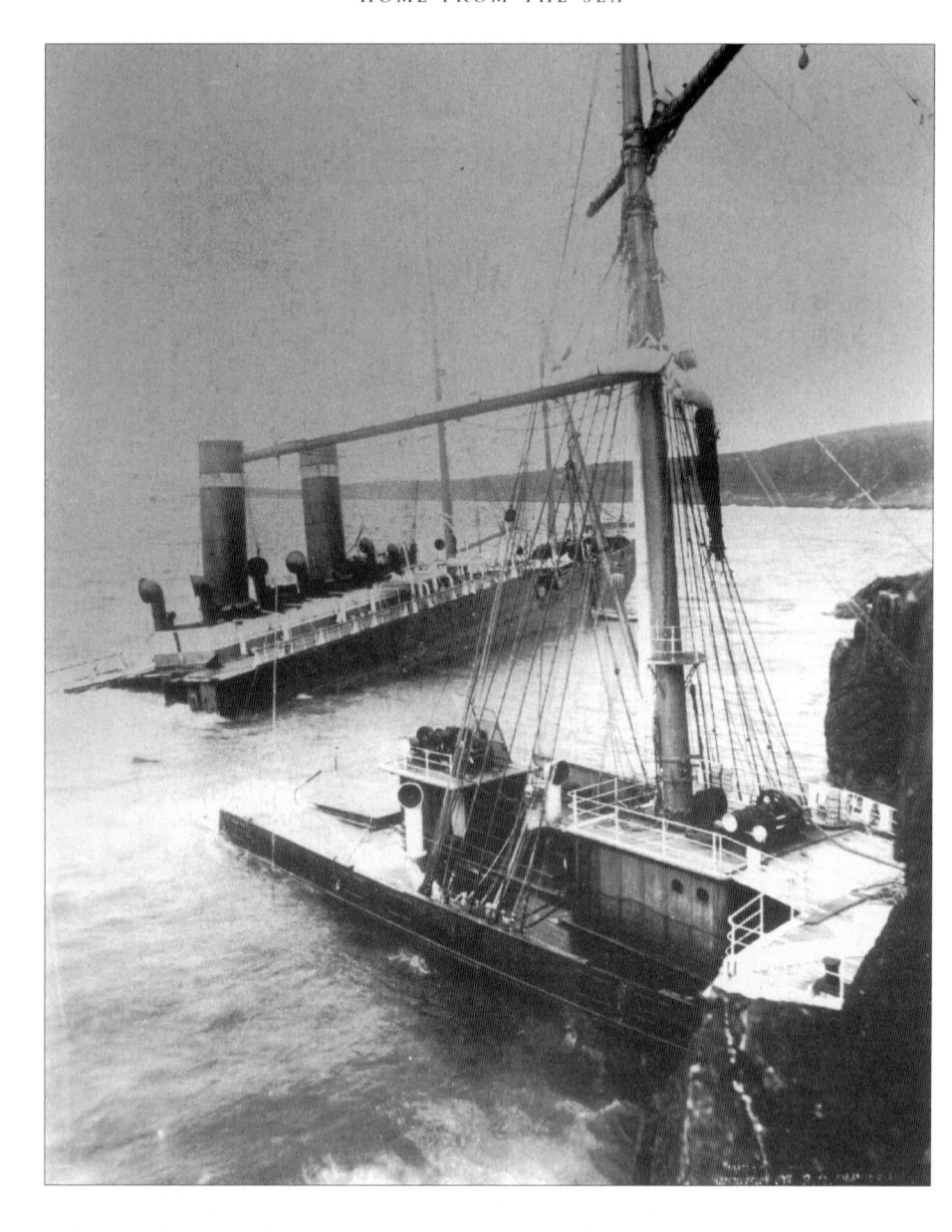

The ***City of Chicago*** after breaking in two before eventually sinking on the Western side of the Old Head of Kinsale in July 1892.

Photograph courtesy of Jonathan Wigham.

CHANGING TIMES

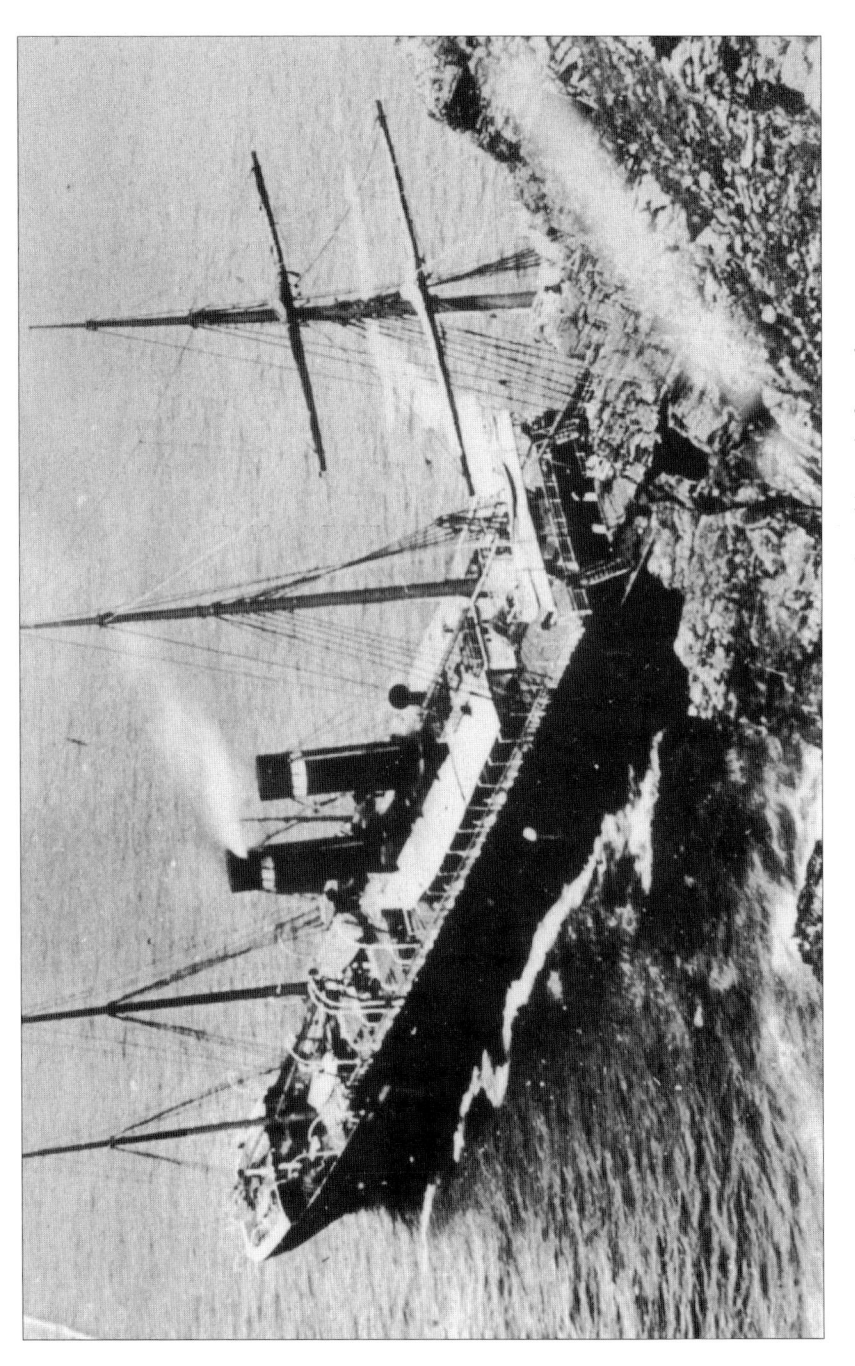

The *City of Chicago* after she had run aground at the Old Head of Kinsale.
Photograph courtesy of Jonathan Wigham.

aground in Dunworley Bay. By now the telephone had arrived in Courtmacsherry and a call was received from Barry's Cove coastguards of the ship's predicament. The Lifeboat launched at 6.00 am and with a willing crew of thirteen aboard they rowed around the Seven Heads to Bird Island where the ship had grounded. The *Ecclefechan* owned by C. T. Guthrie of Glasgow, was carrying a 4,000 tons cargo of grain from San Fransisco to Glasgow.

The Captain was Mr. Jones and he commanded a crew of thirty two. The passage from San Fransisco had taken one hundred and thirty days and having passed the Galley Head the *Ecclefechan*, probably due to the thick fog which enveloped the coast, struck the headland, known as Bird's Island, outside Dunworley Bay. On arrival at Bird's Island, around 8.20 am, the Lifeboat found that the crew of the *Ecclefechan* had taken to the ship's lifeboats and lay alongside, as the ship, though holed, was not in imminent danger of sinking. The *Farrant* returned to Courtmacsherry. The rocket car company had, by now, arrived out on the headland and their assistance was not required either. A gunboat the *Gossamer* tried to tow off the *Ecclefechan* but without success.

Eventually, three tugs from Queenstown, *Mona*, *Flying Fish* and *Flying Fox* arrived under the direction of Ensor Salvage. The three tugs succeeded in towing the stranded ship off and started to tow to Queenstown, soon they discovered that the salvage pumps could not keep pace with the inflow of water.

The *Ecclefechan* was then, immediately, towed to a corner of Dunworley Bay and beached. Over the next few days, temporary repairs were carried out and larger pumps put on board to keep the water under control. The *Ecclefechan* was then towed to Queenstown where she was fully repaired and put back into service.

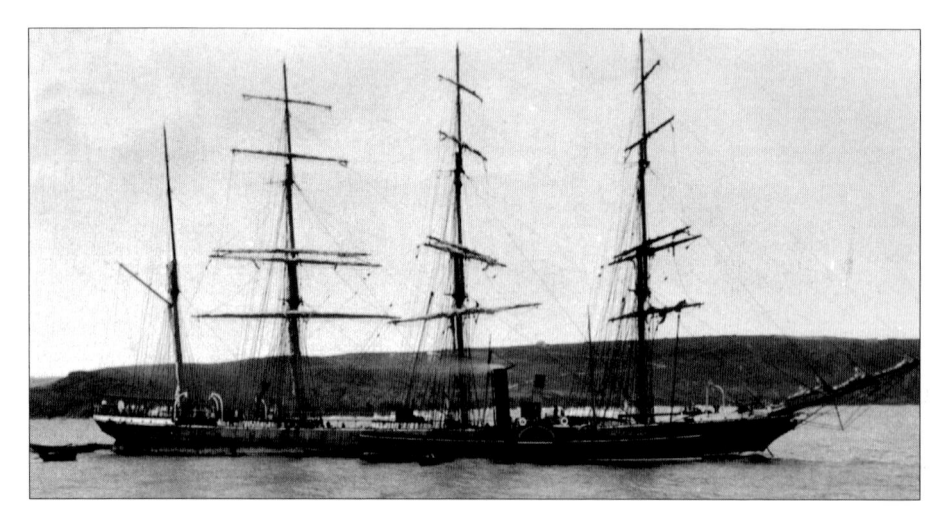

The *Ecclefechan* in Dunworley with Ensor Salvage Tugs standing by.
Photo courtesy of Jonathan Wigham.

CHAPTER 6
MOVING HOUSE
1900 – 1909

> I must go down to the seas again, to the lonely sea and the sky,
> And all I ask is a tall ship and a star to steer her by ,
> And the wheel's kick and the wind's song and the white sail's shaking,
> And a grey mist on the sea's face and a grey dawn breaking.
>
> From 'Sea Fever' by John Masefield (1902)

As a new century dawned the age of steam power in shipping was well and truly upon us. On July 20th 1900, Coxswain Ruddock launched the *Farrant* with a crew of thirteen to go to the aid of a large steamer reportedly in distress at Seven Heads Bay. Launching at 6.00pm they arrived at Seven Heads to find the *Texan*, a 3,000 ton steamer with a thirty man crew, at anchor having been holed in a collision with another ship the *Newton*. The *Texan* was bound from Liverpool to St. Thomas with a general cargo. There

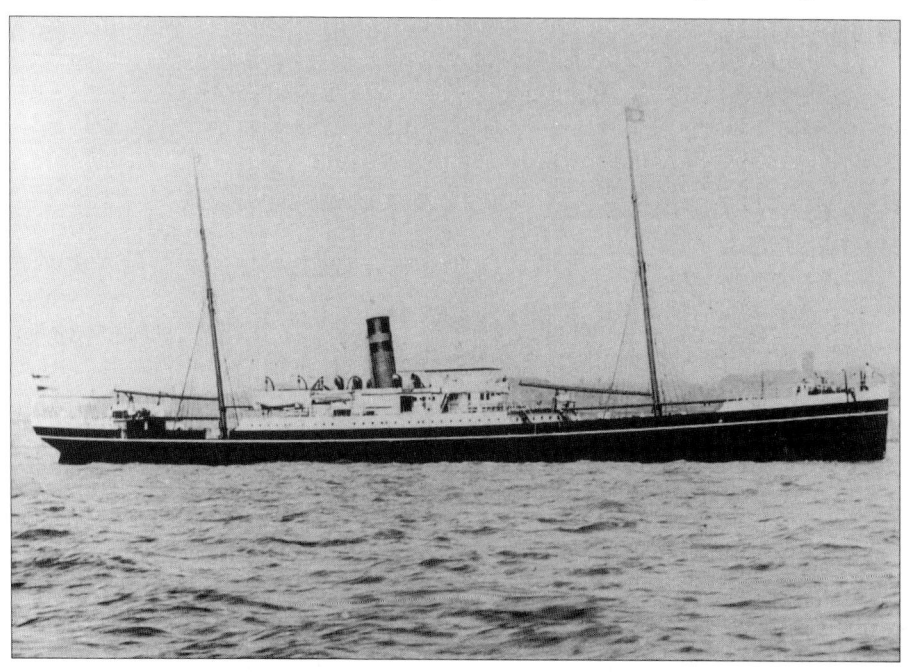

The *Texan* pictured here in Liverpool.
Photo courtesy of the Merseyside Maritime Museum.

was thick fog with a southerly breeze. The Lifeboat remained alongside for some hours as a precaution until the tugboats arrived from Cork returning back to harbour at 1.00am the following morning.

The last service of the **Farrant**, which coincidentally was also the last time the boathouse down at the end of the village (now a private residence) was used, occurred on 14th January 1901. The Lifeboat launched after a report was received that a steamer was drifting ashore just outside the mouth of Courtmacsherry harbour. The Coxswain and crew rowed out past the bar, with a strong gale blowing, but thankfully the steamer had made her way out of the bay safely and the **Farrant** returned to station.
The crew consisted of::-

>   **Noble Ruddock (26)**   **John Donovan (4)**
>   **John Brown (5)**   **John Brien (5)**
>   **James White (3)**   **W. Minihane(-)**
>   **John White(3)**   **J. Foley (5)**
>   **Jer Neil (4)**   **J. Blunt (5)**

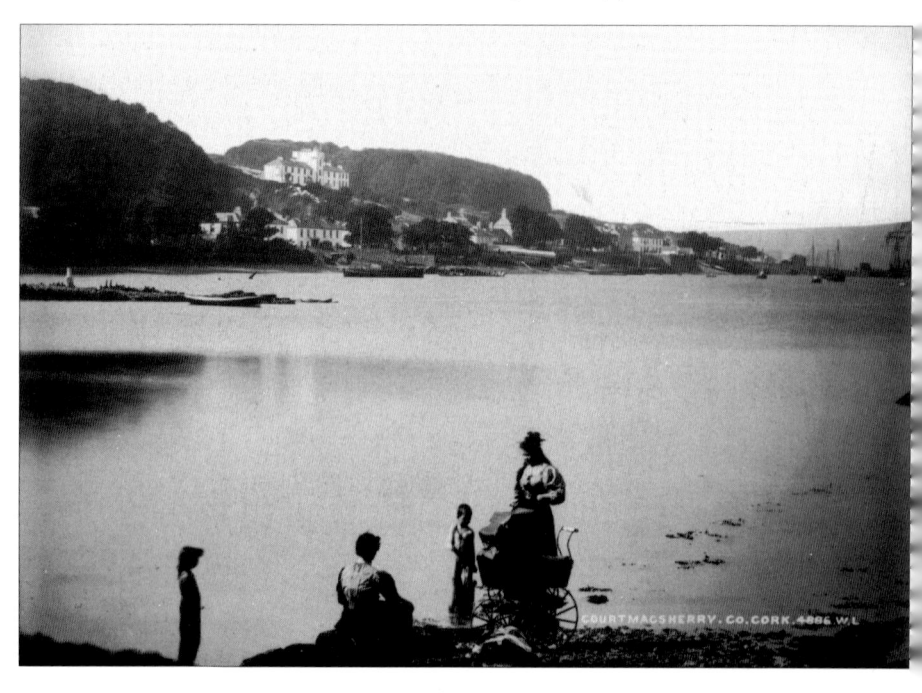

A view of the village taken from the shore beyond the present Hotel.
It is from the famous Lawrence collection taken around the turn of the century.
Photograph courtesy of the National Library of Ireland.

D. Driscoll (-)   M. Holland(1)
J. Mann (4)

Shown in brackets are the number of previous services.

The **Farrant** in her time in Courtmacsherry had launched on service six times and saved six lives. She was sold off that year. The Lifeboat station was relocated to Barry's Point later that year when a new boathouse and slipway was constructed at a cost of £1,300. This consisted of a corrugated iron structure on a concrete base to house the Lifeboat and all the equipment. Also built was a slipway of Karri Timber, 110 feet long on concrete pillars built onto the rocks. (The remains of these pillars can still be seen at low water and the boathouse is now completely altered as a holiday chalet). The new slipway would make it easier to launch and recover the Lifeboat.

On the transfer to Barry's Point a new boat (O.N. 467) was also built, she was a 37 foot long self righter designed for twelve oars and supplied with sails also. Built at a cost of £888 by Thames Ironworks in London, the new boat was funded through a legacy of Mr. A. Gwilt of Norbiton, London and consequently was named **Kezia Gwilt**. The first service of the splendid new craft was on the 7th March, 1902 around 12.30 when the **Kezia Gwilt** travelled across the bay to investigate a report of a vessel in distress but it

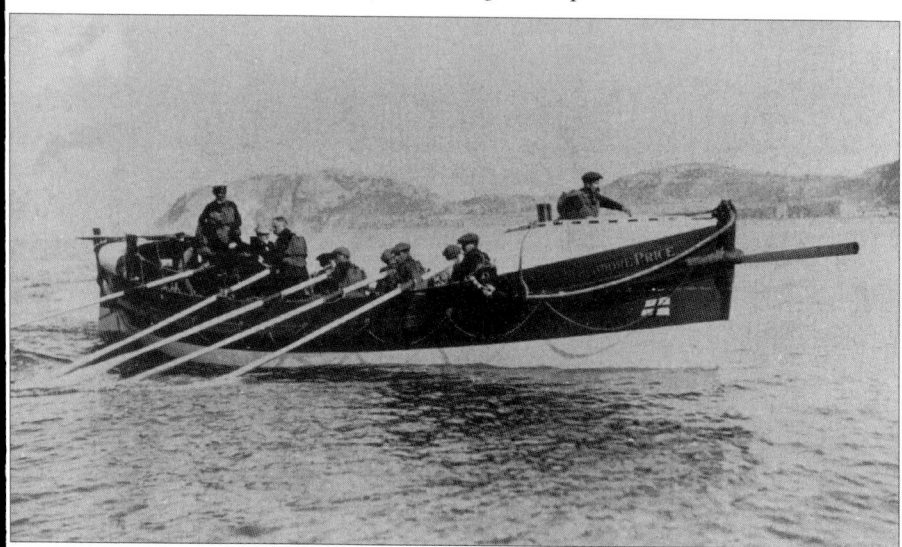

Unfortunately no photograph of the **Kezia Gwilt** seems to exist.
This is the Llandudno Lifeboat **Theodore Price**. She was built a year after the Courtmacsherry boat but the designs were virtually identical.

Photograph courtesy of Llandudno lifeboat

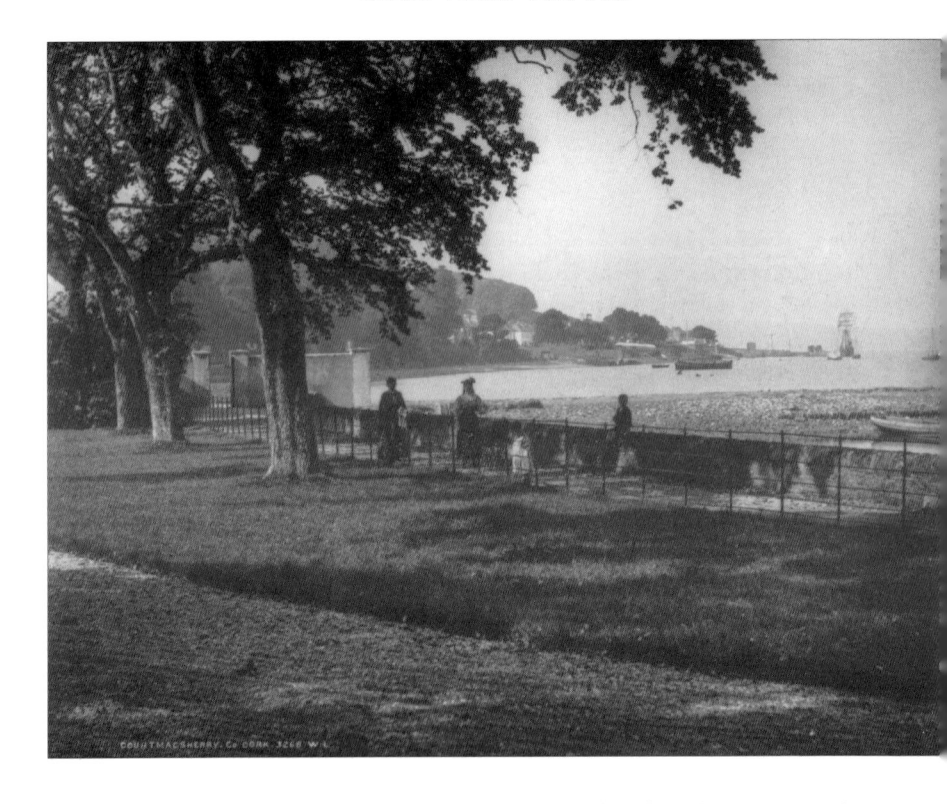

Another Lawrence collection photograph looking up the village from the entrance to the present Hotel. The gate in the background was for pedestrian access along the shore since the present roadway was closed off by a gateway to the private estate of the Earl of Shannon. (now Courtmacsherry Hotel). The small gateway is still visible today.

Photograph courtesy of the National Library of Ireland.

turned out to be a false alarm and the Lifeboat returned to Barry's Point at 4.30pm. Timothy Keohane, the new Coxswain, was on his first service and Rev. Forde, the Rector at Lislee, had now taken over as Hon. Secretary.

A more dramatic service, however, took place on New Year's day 1904. At. 6.30 am on that morning the French Barque **Faulconnier** of Dunkirk carrying 1,715 tons of barley from San Fransisco bound for Queenstown struck the rocks at Travarra. The weather was bad with a strong east-south-east wind and thick haze. A small boat was launched from Travarra cove and took some of the crew of twenty six ashore. On a second run the boat capsized in the rough sea, and all aboard were thrown into the sea although, fortunately they got ashore unharmed. Eleven men still remained on the ship. Courtmacsherry Lifeboat was alerted about 8.00 am and at 8.30 am **Kezia Gwilt** slipped gently into the sea. The fifteen men on board under the command of Tim Keohane, the Coxswain, since

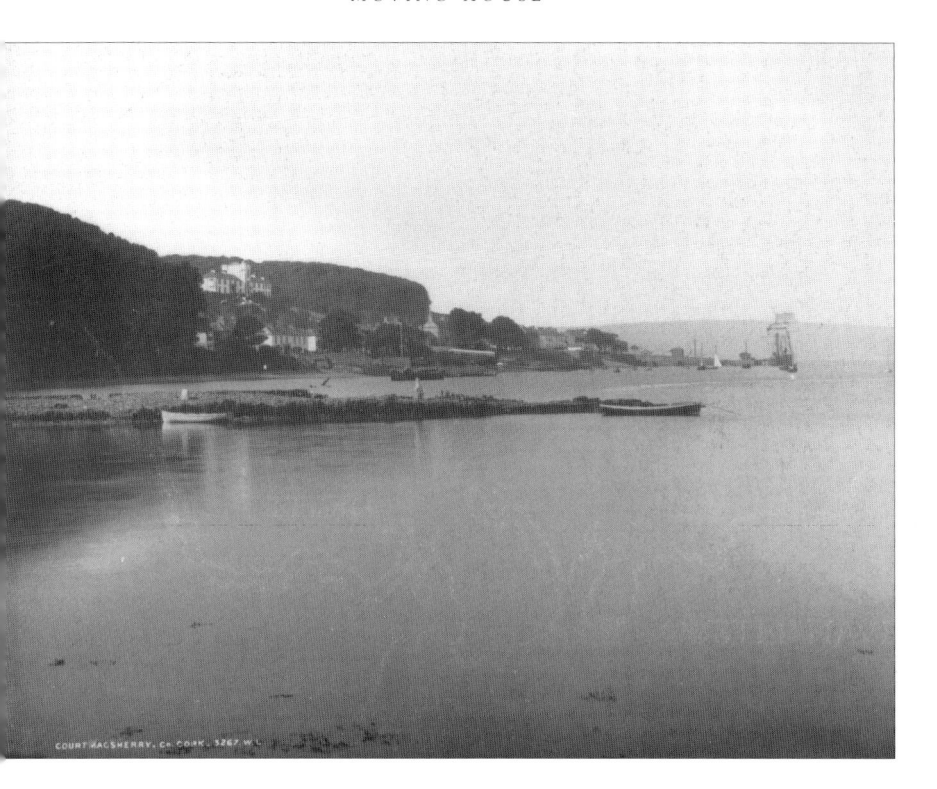

This Lawrence collection photograph shows a sailing ship at the pier and the Coastguard Station having a fine imposing view of the harbour.

Photograph courtesy of the National Library of Ireland.

the transfer to Barry's Point, rowed with urgency around Barry's Point into the teeth of the wind and heavy sea, then southwards for Travarra, arriving on the scene at 9.30 am. The *Faulconnier*, was hard aground with the sea breaking over her. The crew took to their lifeboats but the conditions were too bad to attempt to land ashore. Showing tremendous skill and courage **Kezia Gwilt** was carefully brought alongside the *Faulconnier* and the eleven sailors taken on board. The **Kezia Gwilt** took the men around to Courtmacsherry where they were landed. The Lifeboat then headed back out to Barry's Point where she was rehoused at 3.00 pm.

A tug, the ***Flying Sportsman*** proceeded to Travarra from Queenstown but could not see any hope of saving the vessel and so returned to Queenstown. By Monday the *Faulconnier* had broken in two and became a total loss. It is probable that some local entrepreneurs were able to salvage some pieces from the wreck and a piece of mahogany bearing the ships name came into my possession a few years ago from a local farmer who had been using it as a stick for cattle!

In 1969, a grandson of one of the survivors of that fateful day, Pierre le Garrec, visited Courtmacsherry and Travarra. His grandfather, he reported, though 83 years old, still had clear recollections of his ordeal and the kindness of the people of the Seven Heads and Courtmacsherry.

The **Kezia Gwilt** had a quiet time until November 1908 when she had another false alarm. On this occasion, the Lifeboat was found to have a lot of water on board when hauled up the slip and Rev. Forde urged repairs to be carried out.

Communications in those days were difficult and Rev. Forde pointed out in 1909 that the lack of a direct telegraph line from the coastguard station at the Old Head, to Courtmacsherry was leading to unnecessary delays. Mr. Townshend, his predecessor as Honorary Secretary, had complained of this before in 1891. Yes, indeed, the global village was a long way off then.

CHAPTER 7
THE F.S. CIAMPA
1910 – 1919

> Exultation is the going of an inland soul to sea,
> Past the houses,--past the headlands,--into deep eternity--
> *From Exultation is the going ,by Emily Dickinson 1890.*

A SAD chapter in the coastline of Barryroe was written on the night of 18th February 1910. A terrific gale had been blowing for days causing considerable damage to trees and telegraph lines. Many naval ships of the Atlantic fleet were sheltering in Queenstown. The wind was recorded at sixty five miles an hour from the south-west earlier that evening and the sea was breaking right over the top of Roches Point lighthouse in Cork Harbour. The **F.S. Ciampa**, a barque of 1,400 tons, registered at Castella Maria in Italy, was bravely fighting the storm on her way to Queenstown, with a cargo of nitrates from Mexiolonnes. Now within sight of Queenstown, the journey was soon to come to a tragic conclusion. The **Ciampa**, with a crew of twenty five on board including the master Captain Ostellone, struck Bird Island at Dunworley at 9.00pm. The ill fated ship fired several distress rockets and they were sighted by many locals about 9.30 who then had to travel some distance to telephone the coastguard station at Courtmacsherry.

More travelled out to the rock where the **F.S. Ciampa** perished and, as they got nearer, they heard the pitiful cries of the seamen above the merciless gale. However, when they arrived on the headland which sticks out into the Atlantic, the ship and its crew were gone. The news reached the Honorary Secretary at approximately 10.30pm and a crew was assembled at Barry's Point.

The **Kezia Gwilt** headed off into the boiling cauldron. The fifteen brave crew of the Lifeboat pulled as hard as they could for four miles but could not make any progress against such a storm. Indeed the strain on the oars was so immense that they broke two on the journey. The Lifeboat pulled out to sea in the hope that the wind might moderate and allow them continue but it did not, and **Kezia Gwilt** returned to the Lifeboat house at 8.00am the following morning. Shore help was sent too with rocket carts sent from both Courtmacsherry and Barry's Cove but the same story prevailed, when they arrived nothing was to be seen.

By dawn wreckage and bodies were being washed ashore and the first four bodies were placed in a temporary morgue, in a shed beside Murphy's Pub, in Dunworley. Here on Tuesday morning an inquest was held under Coroner Neville and Rev. Forde, the Honorary Secretary, gave evidence of the Lifeboat's efforts and the fact that

> *The crew were in imminent danger of their lives and did everything that was humanly possible to render assistance to the crew of the ill fated ship.*

Those four bodies were interred in the afternoon at Lislee Cemetery and several more came ashore in the following weeks.

In April of the following year a 2,026 ton steel ship the ***Falls of Garry*** went ashore at Ballymacus Point near Oysterhaven. Although the Lifeboat rowed all the way past the Old Head of Kinsale and on to Oysterhaven, the twenty five crew of the ship had been rescued either by the coastguards, using breeches buoy, or using their own ships lifeboats.

I am sure Coxswain Tim Keohane and crew did not relish the six and a half hour row back against the wind to Barry's Point. In the subsequent years the Lifeboat was launched six more times including the ***Lusitania*** call. The last call of the Lifeboat at Barry's Point, took place on March 14th, 1919 when the coast watcher at Seven Heads mistook the searchlights of a warship as distress signals so the crew of fifteen had a bit of exercise as they rowed out but they were fortunate to be recalled when only two miles gone.

Rev. Forde, the Honorary Secretary, was not in the habit of sparing his words when filling out his report as he records that

> *the coxswain's daughter, when hastening to the boathouse with the recall message,*
> *fell and injured her knee - she is in bed today.*

Her father, Timothy Keohane, had been Coxswain since 1901 and was out on each and every one of the thirteen services during that period.

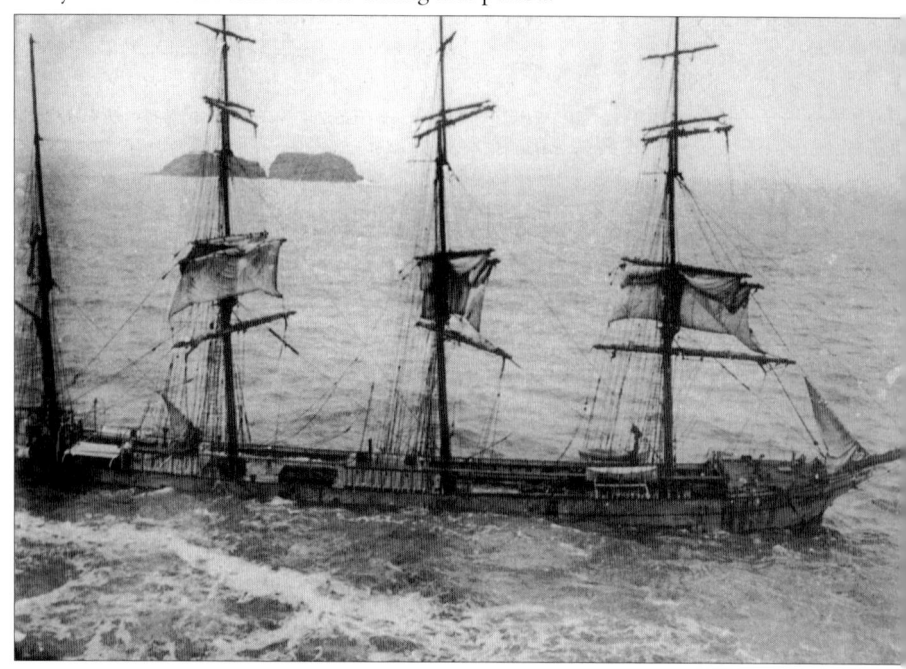

The ***Falls of Garry*** ashore at Ballymacus near Oysterhaven, in the background are the Sovereign Islands.

Photograph courtesy of the Cork Examiner.

CHAPTER 8
THE CARDIFF HALL
1920 – 1929

> Winds whistling thro' the shrouds, proclaim
> A fatal harvest on the deck,
> Quick in pursuit as active flame,
> Too soon the rolling ruin came,
> And ratify' the wreck.
>
> *From Ode on a Storm by William Falconer 1758.*

THE night of the *Cardiff Hall* will be long remembered in the parish of Barryroe for that night saw the havoc of shipwreck upon its shore yet again. On 13th January, 1925, an incredible gale was blowing. Widespread damage was caused all over the south of Ireland including bridges being washed away by floods. Early on in the evening about 6.00pm a ship was sighted at the Seven Heads going eastwards and all looked to be in order. Nothing further was noted until about 8.00pm when the residents of the Seven Heads were startled by the sound of several long blasts of a ships siren above the noise of the storm. The first to go to see what was happening was Patrick Aherne who lived above Travarra, where the men of the *Faulconnier* were rescued some twenty one years earlier.

He saw the lights of a large ship drifting slowly towards land with the siren now blowing continuously. Soon he was joined by more locals and they were soon to see the *Cardiff Hall* go helplessly ashore on the infamous Shoonta Rock outside Travarra cove.

The *Cardiff Hall* was a ship of 3,944 tons, carrying a cargo of maize from Rosario, Riverplate, Argentina to Cork for R and H Hall Limited. The Master was a Welshman, Captain David John Bowen, a seaman of thirty six years experience and he commanded a crew of twenty seven men including his son Trevor who, although only nineteen years of age, was shortly to sit for his Mate's Certificate.

At 8.45pm one of the onlookers went on horseback to Lislevane to telephone for help, the rocket cart from Barry's Cove was summoned and also the Lifeboat station at Barry's Point. Various theories have emerged over the years as to why the Lifeboat did not launch that night. The official records suggest that insufficient men mustered that night which led to the closure of the station in February 1925. This is quite plausible, since what had been a bustling hamlet, some years ago, was by now drastically reduced in numbers. (Today only two people live, permanently, on the headland). Yet the *Cork Examiner* of January 15th reported that:

> *The Lifeboat at Barry's Point was also launched although it was obvious that she would be unable to get around the Point and to attempt to reach the scene would be utterly futile. Nevertheless, a crew stood by in readiness but unfortunately were in the*

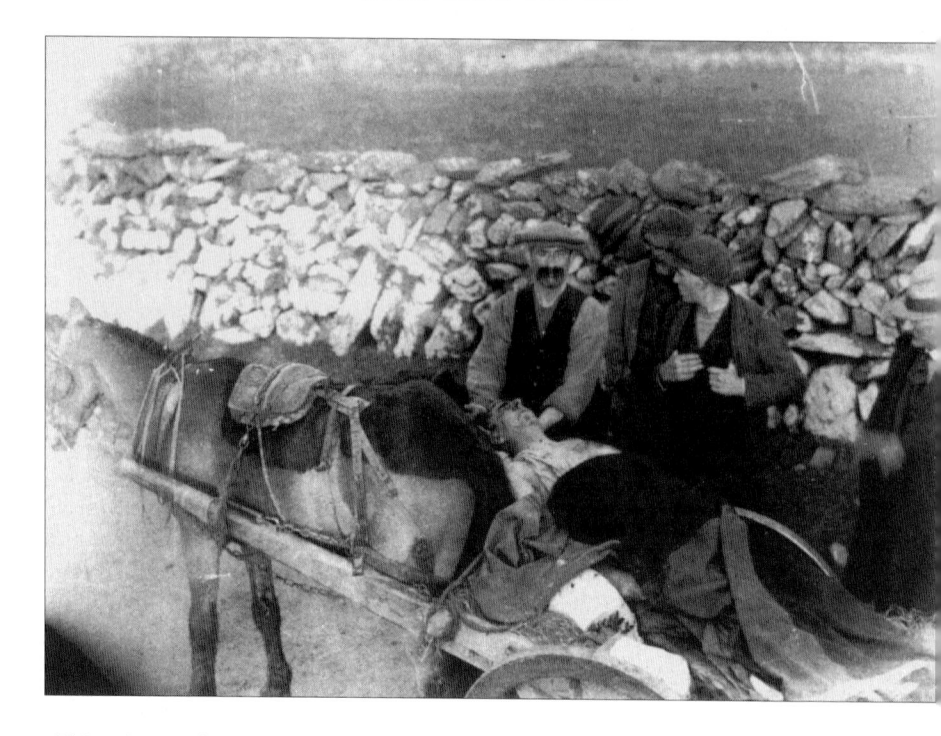

This poignant photograph published in the Cork Examiner Thursday January 15th. 1925 shows the body of Captain Bowen about to be transported to Butlerstown village.
From a copy of the original photograph courtesy of Martin Walsh

> *position of being unable to render assistance. Even if a lifeboat were available at Travarra Bay and was there launched, nothing could be done owing to the position of the wrecked steamer offering no lee shore and to the fact that she broke up in a few minutes.*

Perhaps I shall have to wait to meet all the former crew in that great boathouse in the sky to get an answer!

The rocket cart crew assembled and headed for Travarra arriving at 11.30pm but, by then, it was too late. Within minutes of the doomed ship striking the jagged rocks, she was broken in two and, as the crew screamed for mercy, the **Cardiff Hall** was smashed to pieces and carried them all to their watery grave.

By 9.30pm wreckage was being washed ashore along with the cargo of maize. One piece of the wreck, weighing about two tons, was thrown forty feet above the water's edge onto the mainland. At 10.00pm the grim discovery of the body of Captain Bowen was made, washed ashore only yards, from where, only hours earlier, he commanded such a fine ship. At dawn the cove presented an unusual sight with tons of maize everywhere

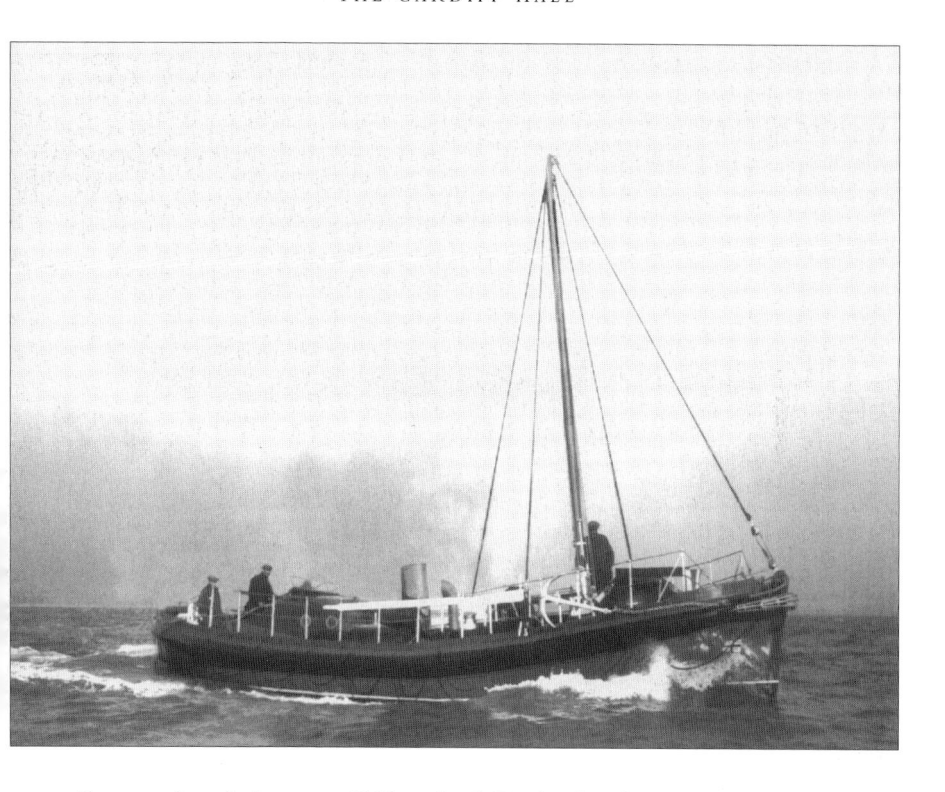

Courtmacsherry's first motor Lifeboat *Sarah Ward and William David Crossweller* on trials off the Isle of Wight.

Photograph courtesy of Beken of Cowes.

and also wreckage of every description. By 10.00am the second and only other body recovered was found by a shore search party. It was of an Arab man about thirty years of age. An inquest was held in Butlerstown on Thursday afternoon and one of those who gave evidence was Paddy Aherne. He told of how he, and others, were powerless to help as they watched the ship flounder below the cliff on which they stood. On Friday afternoon, Captain Bowen's brother, Thomas, and brother in law, Mr. Arthur, arrived in Butlerstown to formally identify his brother's body following which they accompanied his remains back to Wales for burial.

The wreck brought a windfall to the locality as the maize was a very valuable cargo and hundreds of people thronged the cove to recover it and bring it up to the fields to dry it out. Temporary mills were set up in Butlerstown village and buyers came to purchase the maize. The work of trawling more maize up from the bottom of the sea went on for months. All that remains locally of the wreck today is a huge anchor recovered in 1987 by a local diver and now on display near the Community Centre. . . .

... and the stories are still told of the night of the *Cardiff Hall*" . . . . . .

Transfer back to Courtmacsherry.
The station closed temporarily in February 1925 and again in 1928. The following year the first motor Lifeboat was sent to Courtmacsherry.

She was the ***Sarah Ward and William David Crossweller*** (O.N.716) built by J. S. White at a cost of £8,454. A Watson class she was 45 foot 6 inches long, x 12 foot 6 inches wide and powered by two Weyburn CE 4 petrol engines, each of 40 horsepower. This new boat would be a major improvement to the service provided by Courtmacsherry Lifeboat.

The money to pay for this new boat was provided from a legacy of the late Mr. Thomas Crossweller of Kent.

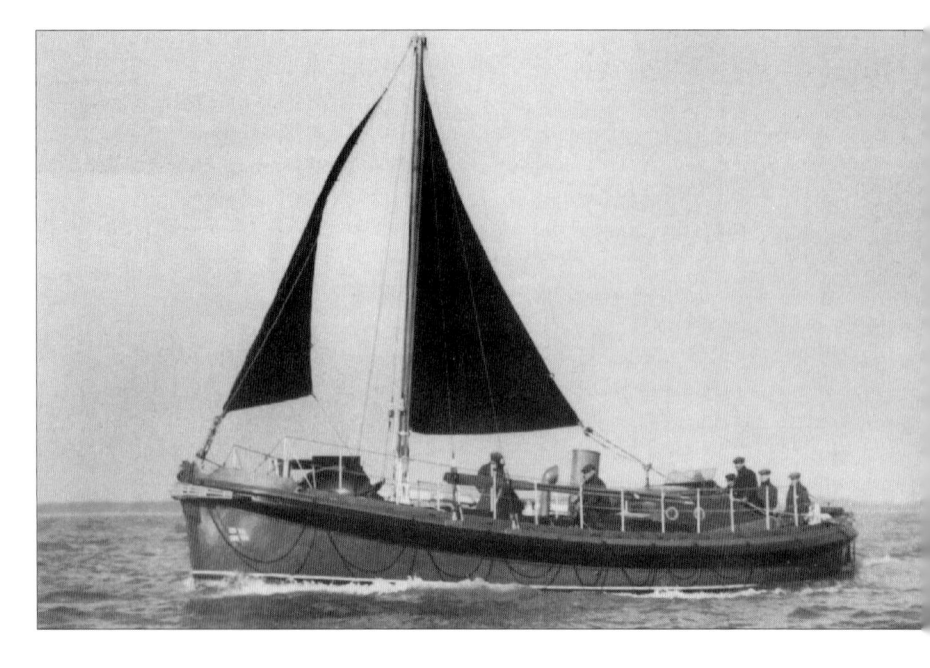

The *Sarah Ward and William David Crossweller* on trials off the Isle of Wight
before coming to Courtmacsherry.
Note that she was fitted with sails as a back up to the petrol engines.
Photograph courtesy of Beken of Cowes.

CHAPTER 9
A PRESIDENTIAL VISIT
1930 – 1939

>The people along the sand
>All turn and look one way.
>They turn their back on the land.
>They look at the sea all day.
>
>*From Neither Out Far Nor In Deep. by Robert Frost 1936.*

WHAT must surely rank as the beginning of a new era for the Courtmacsherry Lifeboat well and truly got underway in the 1930's. To begin with, a Vellum, to record the centenary of the station's establishment, was presented on May 30th, 1930. Present to hand over the parchment to Rev. W.E. White, Chairman of the local committee, was Mr. G. Shee, Secretary of the R.N.L.I. who had travelled from London to make the presentation. The magnificent new motor Lifeboat was now stationed at anchor in Courtmacsherry harbour and ready for her first call to service. ***Sarah Ward and William David Crossweller*** had to wait until 27th October, 1930 before that call came. The new crew had an uneventful search for a steam trawler four miles south-east of the Galley Head, spending over five hours at sea.

The coxswain was Thomas Bulpin, an experienced seaman, who having sailed many times into Courtmacsherry, married a local girl and settled here.

The first motor mechanic was **Percy Egan** who had served as engineer on many ships before coming to Courtmacsherry. The rest of the inaugural crew were :-

>*Denis Whelton*   *Denis Driscoll*
>*D. White*   *M. Dempsey*
>*T. Brown*   *H. Jeffers*
>*James Whelton* (affectionately known as '90')

Also on board was **Noble Ruddock** the Hon Secretary's nephew who eventually went on to serve the R.N.L.I. as District Engineer for Ireland.

The Naming Ceremony.

Monday July 6th, 1931 brought a huge crowd to Courtmacsherry to witness the naming ceremony of ***Sarah Ward and William David Crossweller***. The village was spruced up from end to end including an archway of flowers over the roadway at the entrance to the village and a banner proclaiming *Céad Míle Fáilte* to the arriving visitors and dignitaries. Several boats made the trip around from Cork harbour to add spectacle to the scene.

Rev. W.E. White, President of the Courtmacsherry branch of the Institution, who presided, reminded his listeners that they were there to inaugurate the presentation of the

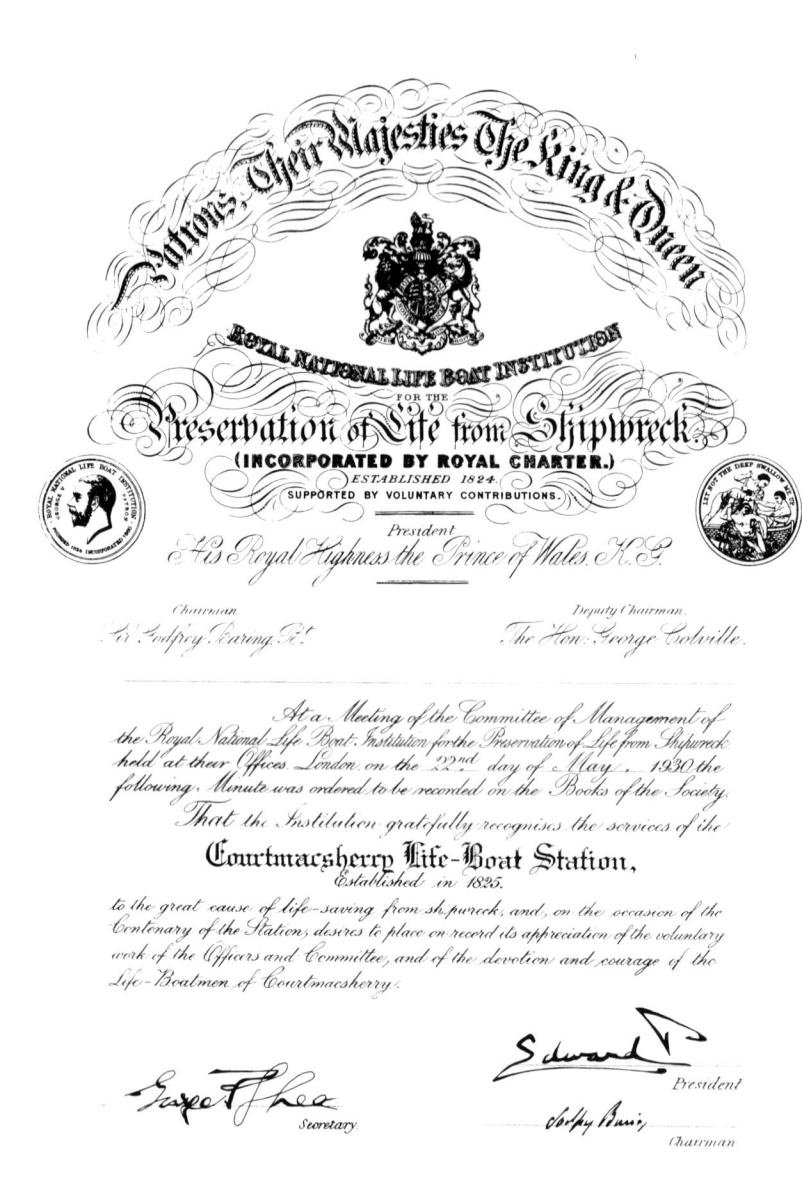

> Patrons, Their Majesties The King & Queen
>
> ROYAL NATIONAL LIFE BOAT INSTITUTION
> FOR THE
> Preservation of Life from Shipwreck
> (INCORPORATED BY ROYAL CHARTER.)
> ESTABLISHED 1824
> SUPPORTED BY VOLUNTARY CONTRIBUTIONS
>
> *President*
> His Royal Highness the Prince of Wales, K.G.
>
> *Chairman*   *Deputy Chairman*
> Sir Godfrey Baring, Bt.   The Hon. George Colville
>
> At a Meeting of the Committee of Management of the Royal National Life-Boat Institution for the Preservation of Life from Shipwreck, held at their Offices, London, on the 22nd day of May, 1930 the following Minute was ordered to be recorded on the Books of the Society.
>
> That the Institution gratefully recognises the services of the
>
> **Courtmacsherry Life-Boat Station,**
> Established in 1825.
>
> to the great cause of life-saving from shipwreck, and, on the occasion of the Centenary of the Station, desires to place on record its appreciation of the voluntary work of the Officers and Committee, and of the devotion and courage of the Life-Boatmen of Courtmacsherry.
>
> Edward   *President*
> George Shee   *Secretary*
> Godfrey Baring   *Chairman*

This is the Centenary Vellum presented to Coutrmacsherry Lifeboat Station on Friday May 30th 1930. The Vellum was presented by Mr. George Shee Secretary of the RNLI, to Rev. E. White, Chairman of the local branch.

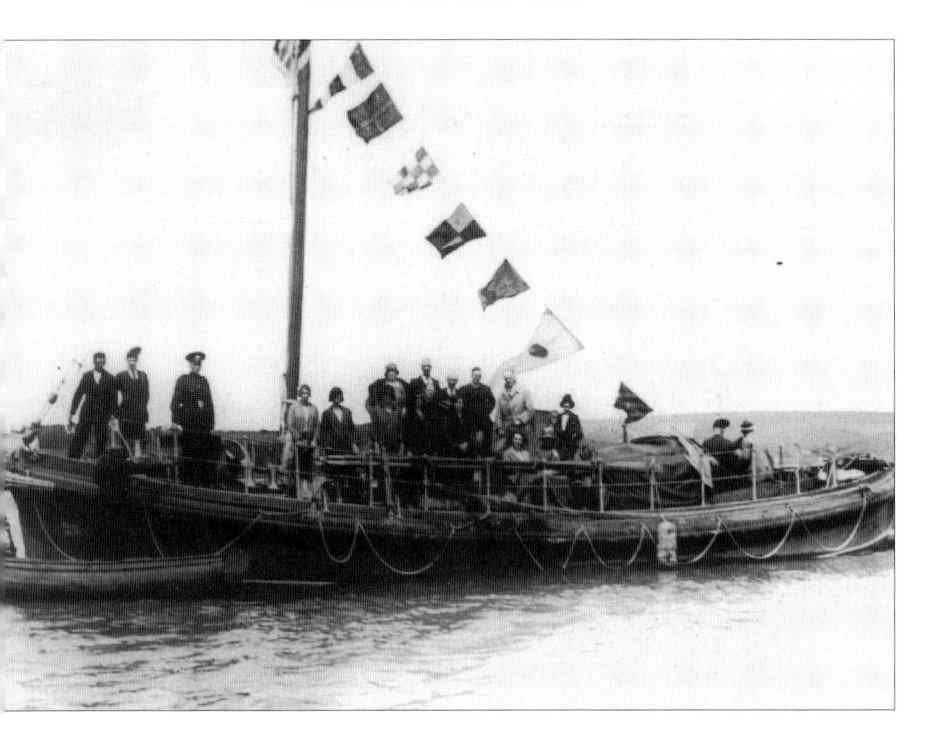

A group pictured aboard the Lifeboat on Friday May 30th. 1930 following the presentation of the Centenary Vellum.

Photograph courtesy of the Cork Examiner.

Lifeboat and it's dedication to the glory of God and the service of humanity. Commander E.D. Drury, Chief Inspector of Lifeboats, gave a full description of the Lifeboat mentioning that in fine weather she could carry at least one hundred and twenty and in rough weather about ninety. The underdeck part of the boat was divided into eight watertight compartments which contained about one hundred and fifty air spaces. She was equipped with a gun capable of throwing a line about eighty yards. He congratulated the Courtmacsherry station on it's efficiency and good record.

Rear Admiral, T.P.M. Beamish, M.P., a member of the R.N.L.I. Committee of Management, spoke, and amongst his remarks, he said that the Courtmacsherry boat had been out thirty six times and had saved thirty nine lives.

The Barryroe Church Choir sang some hymns before Mrs. Cosgrave, wife of the President of Ireland, stepped forward to formally name the Lifeboat ***Sarah Ward and William David Crossweller,*** in memory of the late Mr.Thomas Crossweller of Sidcup, Kent, donor of the legacy out of which the cost was defrayed:

I name this lifeboat Sarah Ward and William David Crossweller and I pray that

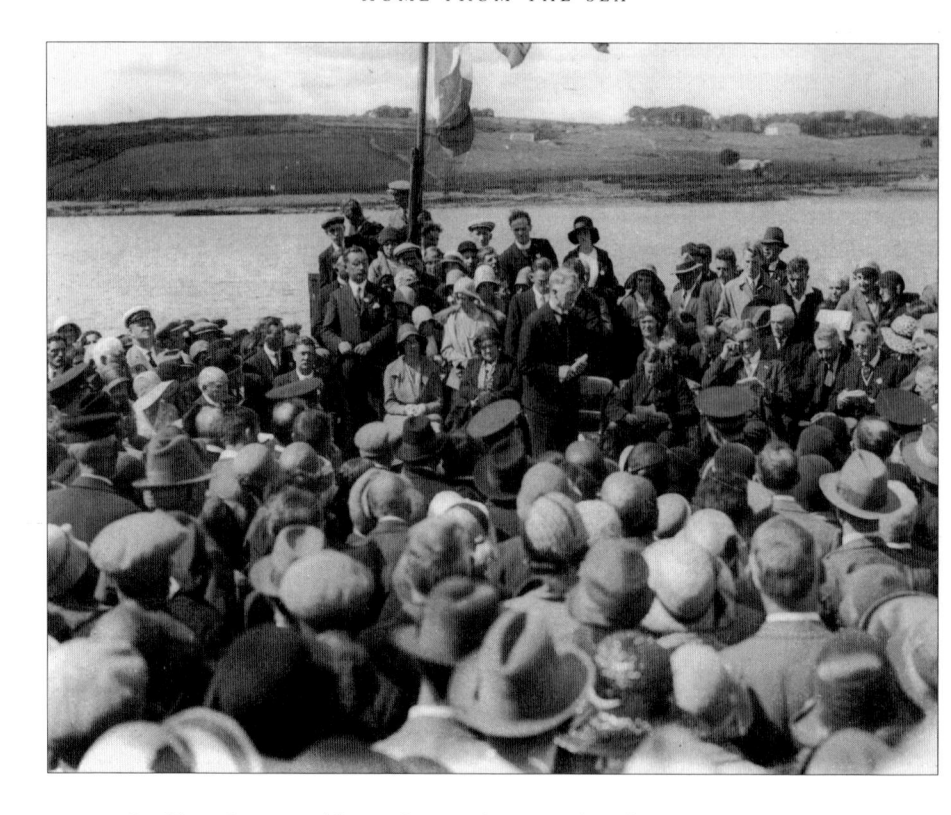

President Cosgrave addresses the crowd prior to the official naming and blessing of ***Sarah Ward and William David Crossweller*** on Monday July 6th.1931.
Photograph courtesy of the Cork Examiner.

she may go on her errand of mercy with the blessing of almighty God and the good wishes of the Irish people .

President
spoke at length on the great work of the Lifeboats around the coast and of the support it receives from people everywhere. Also among the large number of dignitaries that attended were Mr. T. J. O'Donovan, T.D., Mr. J. T. Wolfe, T.D., Mr. T. Sheehy, T.D., and Mr. T. J. Murphy, T.D. who on addressing the crowd perhaps reflecting on the recent turmoil in the country said :

Though they differed in other matters it was a pleasure to find that there were some things on which they could unite on a common platform

Music for the occasion was provided by the No.2 Army band and hymns were sung by the Barryroe Church choir. A memorable day indeed and it was the only time such a major Lifeboat ceremony had taken place in the village and we are glad to be here in 1995

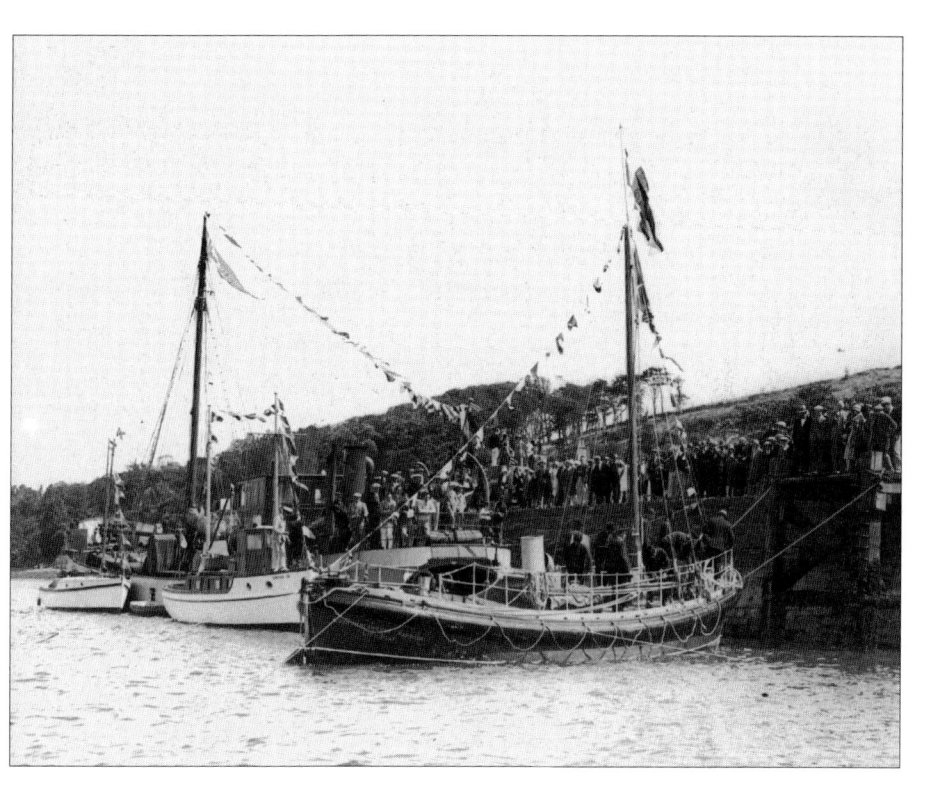

The lifeboat moored outside the pier for the naming ceremony, with a small coaster and visiting boats also at the pier.

Photograph courtesy of the Cork Examiner.

for the next.

A rescue which tested the mettle of the Lifeboat and crew occurred in December of the following year. On Thursday 8th December, 1932, a church holiday, a dance was in full swing in the village at 10.30pm when the call came that a vessel was in distress off Garrettstown strand. As the *Examiner* report of the Saturday recounts:

> *some of the crew, Captain Bulpin who among his other seafaring attributes is an outstanding performer on the concertina, were at the dance, but the sudden call to duty quickly changed the atmosphere of pleasure and merrymaking to one of strain and anxiety as the gallant crew rushed to their station to man their boat and put forth in the face of terrible danger, risking all, to save the lives of their fellow men in distress.*

The **Elizabeth Drew**, a schooner of 180 tons, had left Milford Haven in Wales on Monday bound for Devon and had nearly reached Lands End by Tuesday. The wind then

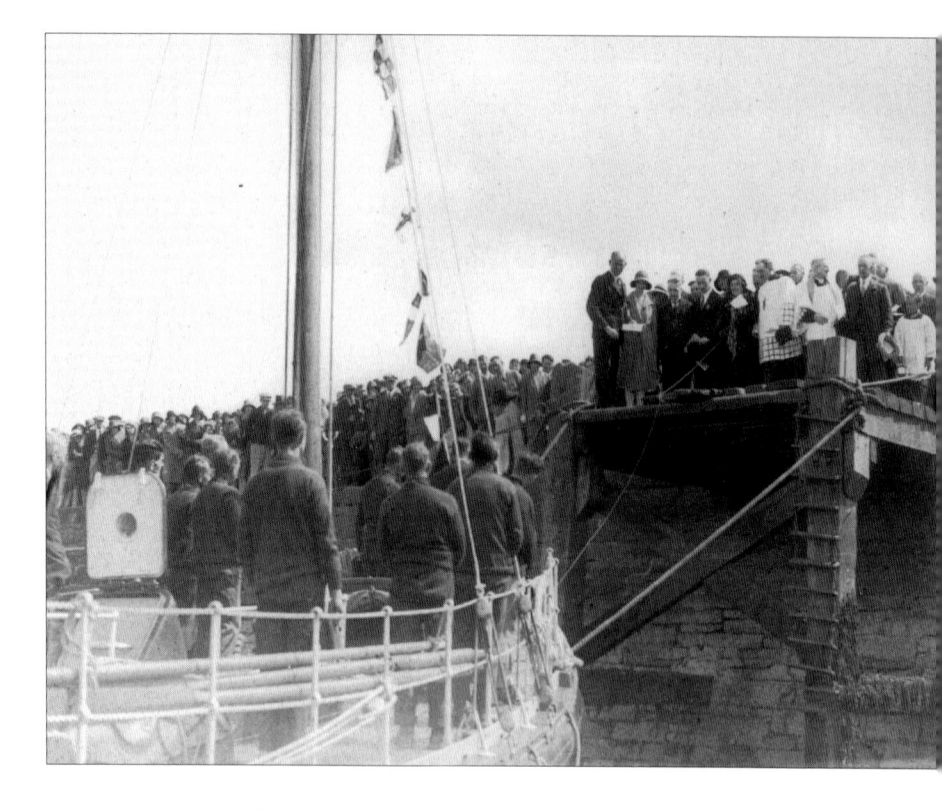

Mrs Cosgrave wife of the President of Ireland steps out onto the small jetty to officially name the new lifeboat on Monday July 6th. 1931.

Photograph courtesy of the Cork Examiner.

freshened so much that the ship could make no headway. The small auxiliary engine was started but could do nothing either against the heavy sea before it eventually failed.

The sails now having been blown out the **Elizabeth Drew** was at the mercy of the east-south-east gale and drifted helplessly north west all day Tuesday and Wednesday firing distress rockets on Tuesday night. The schooner arrived off the Old Head of Kinsale on Thursday evening and Thomas Roones, the Captain, knowing the coast well, as he had often sailed in and out of Courtmacsherry, decided to put up a temporary sail and sail under the shelter of the Old Head of Kinsale and anchor.

They fired distress rockets at 9.30 pm and were delighted to see the **Sarah Ward and William David Crossweller** coming towards them at 11.15pm. The Lifeboat stood by the stricken vessel and poured oil on the raging sea to give the schooner's crew a chance to repair their engine. After two hours work the **Elizabeth Drew's** engine spurted into life and she slipped her anchor and escorted by the lifeboat, crossed the bar into

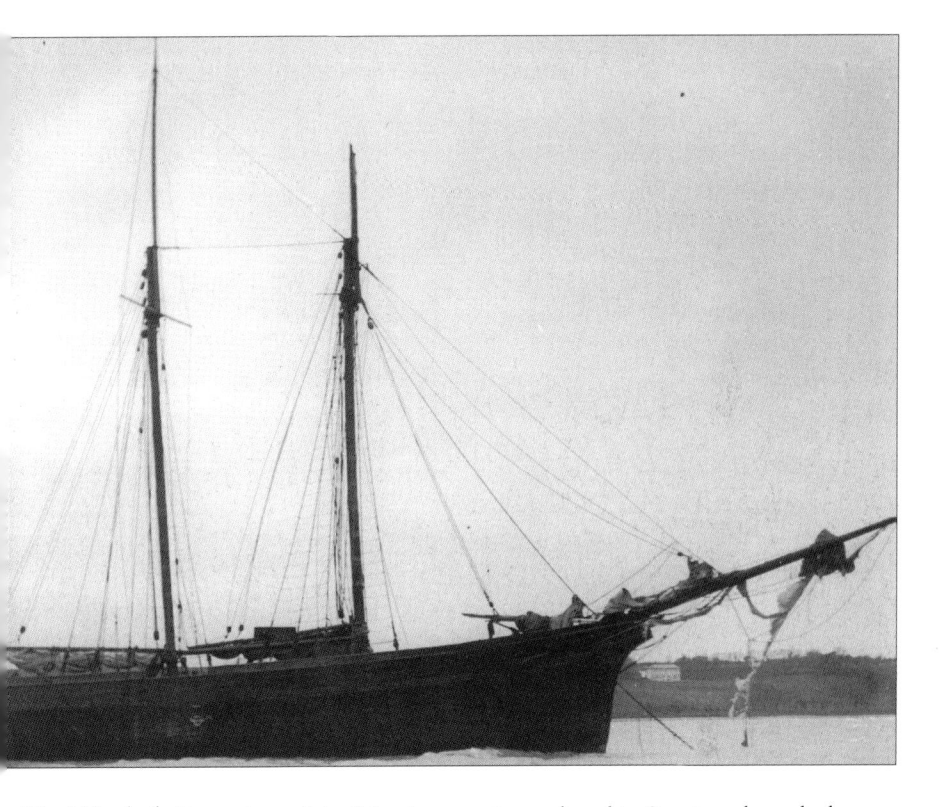

The **Elizabeth Drew** pictured the following morning anchored in Courtmacsherry harbour.
The damage to the rigging of the ship can be clearly seen.
Photograph courtesy of the Cork Examiner.

Courtmacsherry Harbour about 2.00am while the Lifeboat poured more oil onto the sea at the harbour mouth. In typical Lifeboat men fashion, who never lose out on a party, the *Cork Examiner* report further stated that:

> *After a very splendid achievement Captain Bulpin and his men with typical seafaring insouciance forthwith returned to the interrupted pleasures of the dance.*

On the 24th of June 1938 a 200 ton Spanish trawler the **Baron of Vigo** ran aground at the Old Head of Kinsale in thick fog. Luckily the weather was calm, however the impact put a large gash in the trawler's hull and she began to sink slowly. The **Baron of Vigo** kept hooting her siren and soon two local fishermen from the Old Head of Kinsale were on the scene. The lifesaving unit from the Old Head also arrived to render assistance and they in turn summoned the Lifeboat from Courtmacsherry. **Sarah Ward and William David Crossweller** arrived at 4 a.m, by that time however a sister ship of the Baron's was standing by and was transferring the gear off the stricken trawler. As the tide dropped the

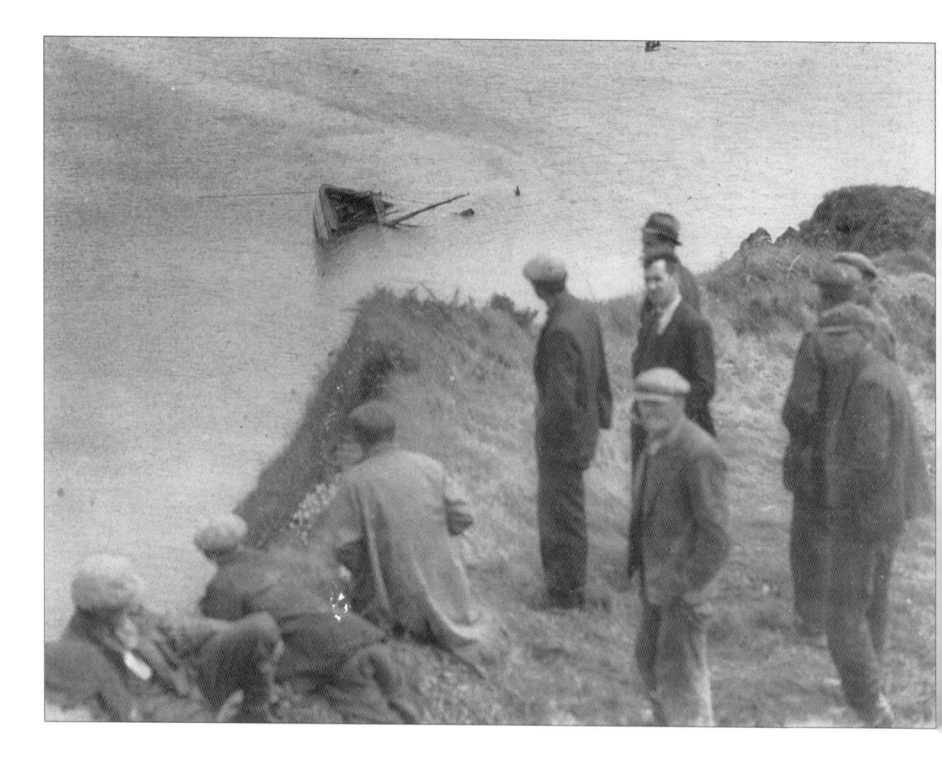

The ***Baron of Vigo*** almost completely submerged after striking the Old Head of Kinsale in thick fog on the 24th. of June 1936.

Photograph courtesy of the Cork Examiner.

trawler developed a list on the rocks and eventually sank.

Ireland was rebuilding itself after many difficult years but the storm clouds of war were gathering in Europe and the eventual onset of hostilities in 1939 brought a very busy time for lifeboats. The threat to shipping by U-boats, especially, kept Courtmacsherry Lifeboat active during these years. On the morning of Friday 15th September 1939, the Lifeboat put to sea to rendezvous with a Norwegian ship the ***Ida Bakke***. She was on her way to the U.S. and was requested to stop by a German submarine which had sunk an oil tanker called the ***British Influence*** carrying over 12,000 tons of fuel on Thursday. The U-boat commander had allowed the ***British Influence*** s crew of forty two to take to their lifeboats before firing a torpedo to sink it, he then stood by for five hours until the ***Ida Bakke*** was sighted and took the crew on board. They were then approximately two hundred miles off the Fastnet.

The Norwegian ship had to return East to meet ***Sarah Ward and William David Crossweller*** off the Old Head of Kinsale where the men were transferred and landed at Courtmacsherry. The unfortunate mariners were, it seems, well looked after in

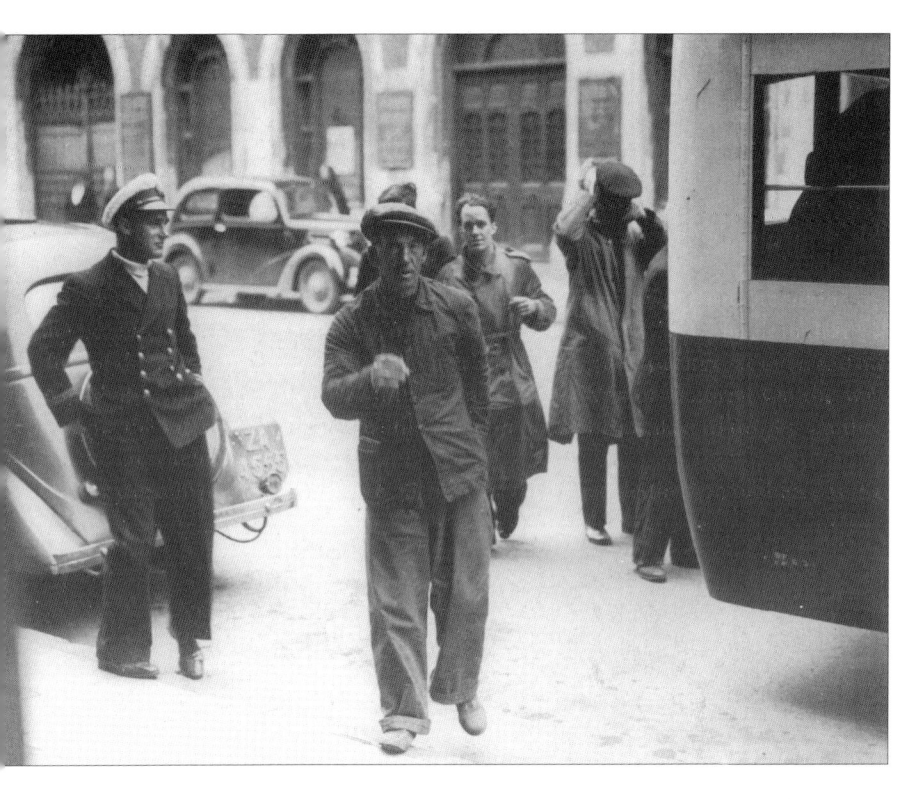

The crew of the **British Influence** pictured at Cork city following their arrival by bus from Courtmacsherry

Photograph courtesy of the Cork Examiner.

Courtmacsherry, before a bus took them to Cork City since the second engineer, Norman Ray, reported that :

> The people of Courtmacsherry nearly killed us with kindness. The Lifeboat Committee and nearly every resident of the town were waiting for us and as the men came ashore different people took groups of them to their homes and gave them hot tea and drinks .

On the following day another ship was sunk by submarine off the Fastnet.

This ship was again an oil tanker the **S.S. Cheyenne** of 8,800 tons. By providence the **Ida Bakke** was again nearby and brought the thirty seven crew back towards the Irish coast and met Courtmacsherry Lifeboat off the Mizen Head about 6.00 am Saturday morning and transferred the survivors to them. The Baltimore Lifeboat was off service for her annual overhaul which is why the Courtmacsherry boat travelled so far west. (It was not the practice to have relief Lifeboats at station in those days) The Master of the

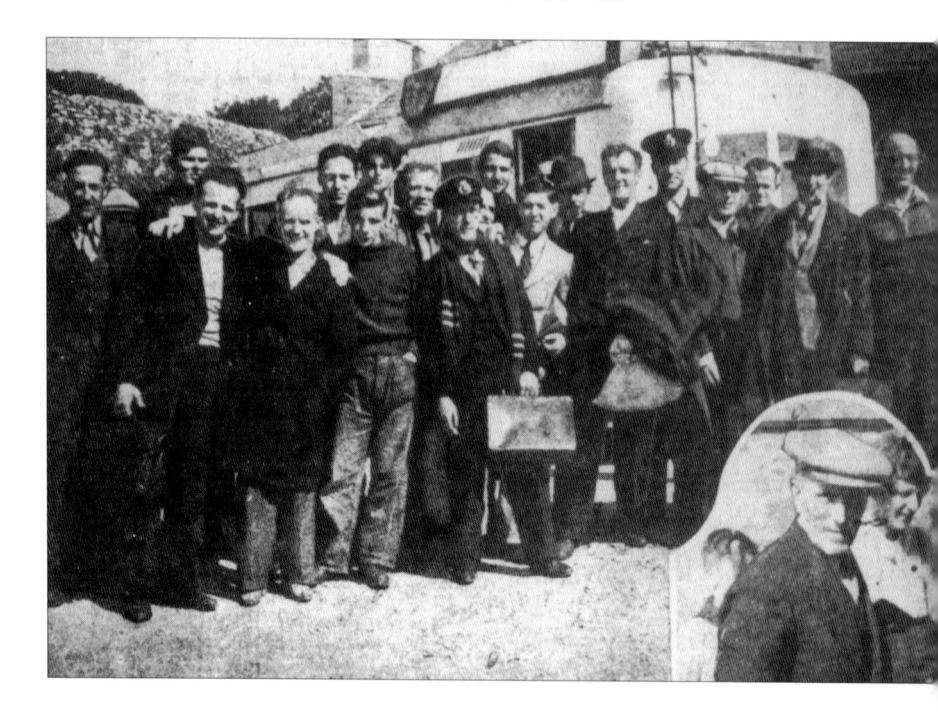

The crew of the ***Cheyenne*** about to board the bus at Baltimore for Cork having been brought ashore by Courtmacsherry lifeboat. In spite of their ordeal they seem to be cheerful enough! Inset is the master of the ***Cheyenne*** Captain Hugh Kerr of Belfast.

Photograph courtesy of the Cork Examiner.

Ida Bakke remarked that - if this kept up he would never reach America! ***Sarah Ward and William David Crossweller*** landed the thirty seven men at Baltimore before returning to Courtmacsherry.

Another long distance trip occurred eight days later, on the 24th of September ***Sarah Ward and William David Crossweller*** had to carry out a search South of Cape Clear and West as far as the Mizen Head. The cargo ship ***S.S. Hayleside*** was sunk by a torpedo fired by a U boat. An extensive search was carried out by the Lifeboat but a local boat had picked up the survivors and landed them in Schull.

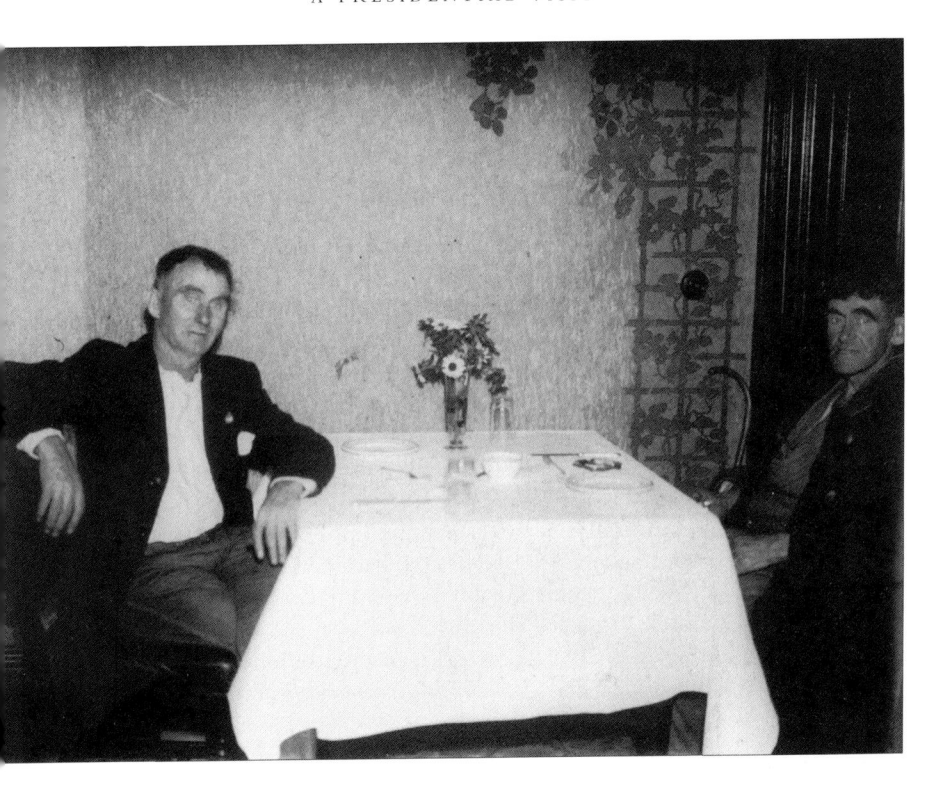

Two of the rescued crew of the ***British Influence*** awaiting a well deserved meal in a Cork city hotel following their arrival from Courtmacsherry.
Photograph courtesy of the Cork Examiner.

CHAPTER 10
THE PERILS OF WAR
1940 – 1949

> The watch changes and changes
> Again. We edge through a minefield,
> Real or imaginary. The speed of the convoy
> Is the speed of the slowest ship.
> *From Night Patrol by Alan Ross 1954.*

As the war continued the U-Boat menace continued with further sinkings off the Cork coast. The war brought a temporary halt to the holiday railway excursions to the village from Cork and Bandon and this, coupled with the general shortages, made for a bleak time locally.

The Lifeboat had several searches for drifting ships lifeboats during 1940 but the danger to shipping was not confined solely to submarines. On the 2nd. December, 1940 a British trawler, the **S.S. Kilgerran Castle**, was bombed by a German plane twenty five miles off the Old Head of Kinsale. The trawler was engulfed in flames and the crew of ten had to take to their lifeboats. Luckily, other trawlers were in the area and picked up the crew so when **Sarah Ward and David William Crossweller** arrived on the scene, their assistance was not required.

Towards the end of the war, the largest number of survivors ever carried by a Courtmacsherry Lifeboat were landed at Courtmacsherry. It all began off the Galley Head during the early morning of March 13, 1945 when distress signals were sighted. A German submarine (U-260), probably knowing the war was nearly at an end, apparently scuttled their ship off the Galley Head and the crew of forty eight took to their liferafts.

Courtmacsherry Lifeboat arrived on the scene about 8.40am and took thirty seven men on board. The other eleven had got safely onto the rocks at the Galley Head and were taken into custody by the Irish army, since Ireland was neutral during the war. When arriving back into harbour, **Sarah Ward and David William Crossweller** was well laden.

The Irish army were out in strength there as well, to line the shore and take the hapless Germans into custody and join their comrades to be interned, at the Curragh, until the end of the war. The Commander of the submarine, reportedly, gave his Luger revolver to Denis Whelton, the 2nd. Coxswain, as a momento, but when word got out, the Garda came to recover it a few days later.

Due to a Government censorship at the time no mention of the rescue, or any photograph, appeared in the newspapers of the time. The first mention of the event was not until the 12th May when censorship was lifted on cessation of the State of Emergency originally declared in 1939. That service marked the end of war related activities and the normal pattern of services kept the Lifeboat busy throughout the following years.

THE PERILS OF WAR

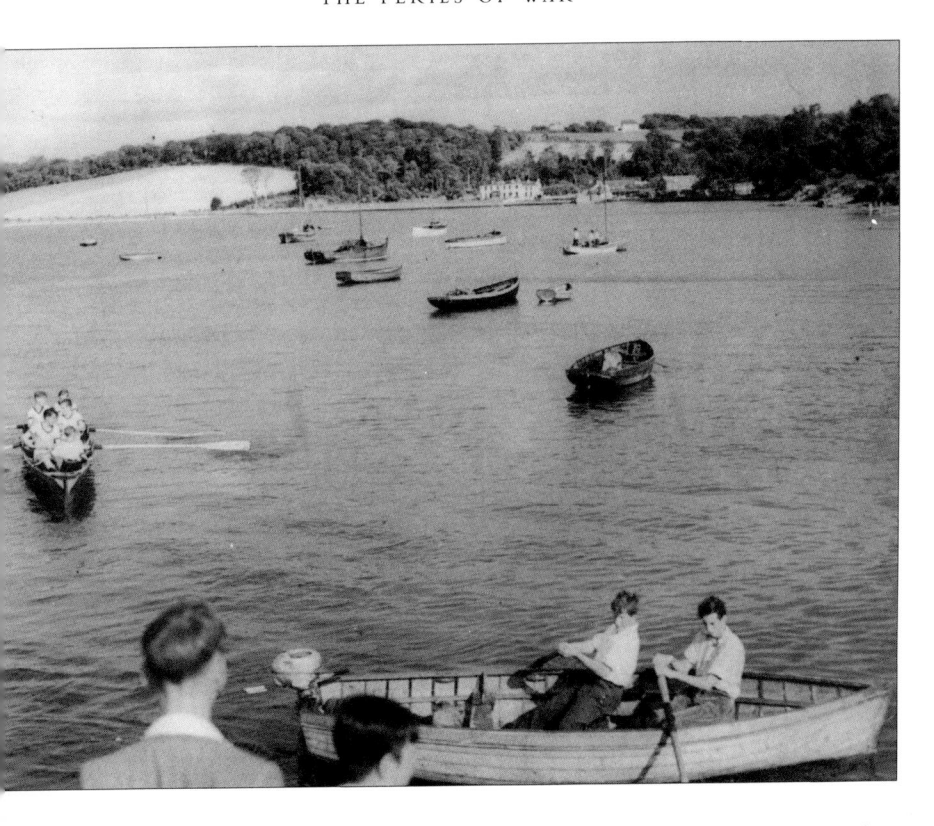

A green field in the back ground where the caravan park and several more houses now stand. This photograph was taken in August 1955.

Photograph courtesy of the Cork Examiner.

CHAPTER 11
A FOND FAREWELL
1950 – 1959

In midst of dangers, fears and death,
Thy goodness I'll adore,
And praise thee for thy mercies past;
And humbly hope for more.

From a letter to The Spectator by Joseph Addison. 1712

THE uncertainty of the Second World War had been left behind and the country was getting back to normal. The excursion trains from Cork had recommenced. Eighteen new Council Houses were built to replace the small cottages at Siberia. Changes

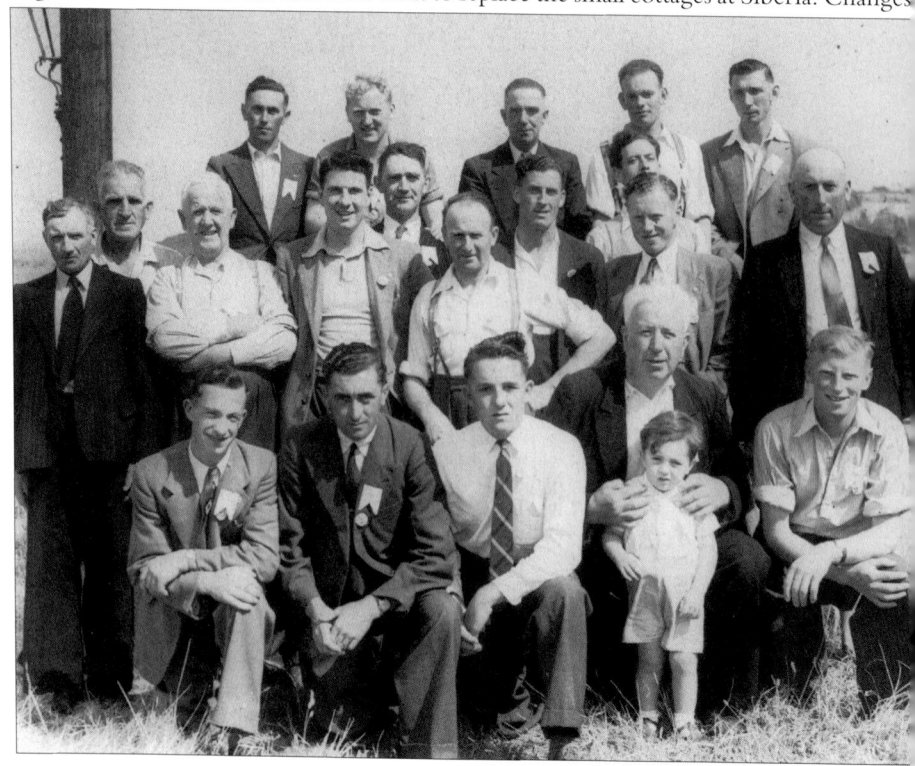

The Regatta Committee pictured on Thursday August 4th. 1955.
Picture courtesy of the Cork Examiner

48

A FOND FAREWELL

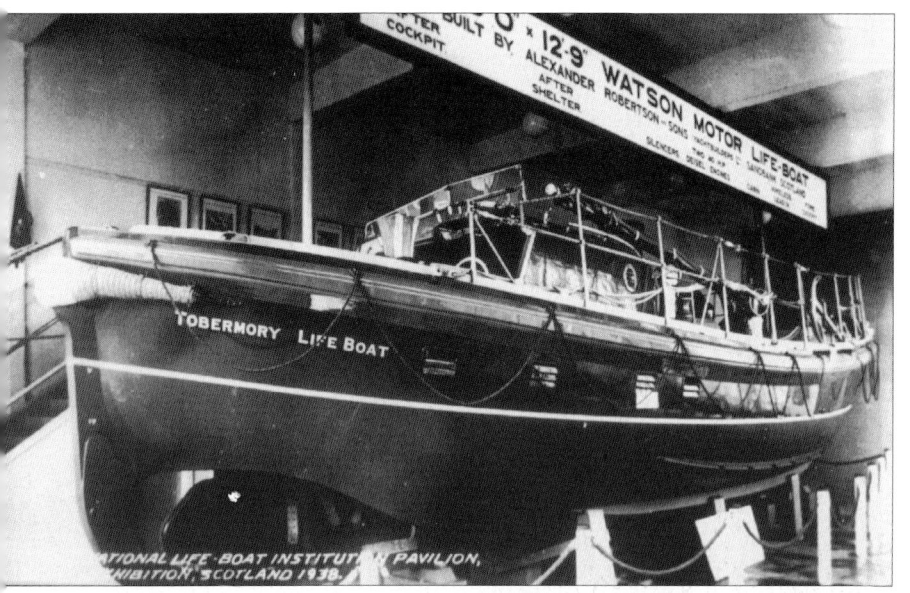

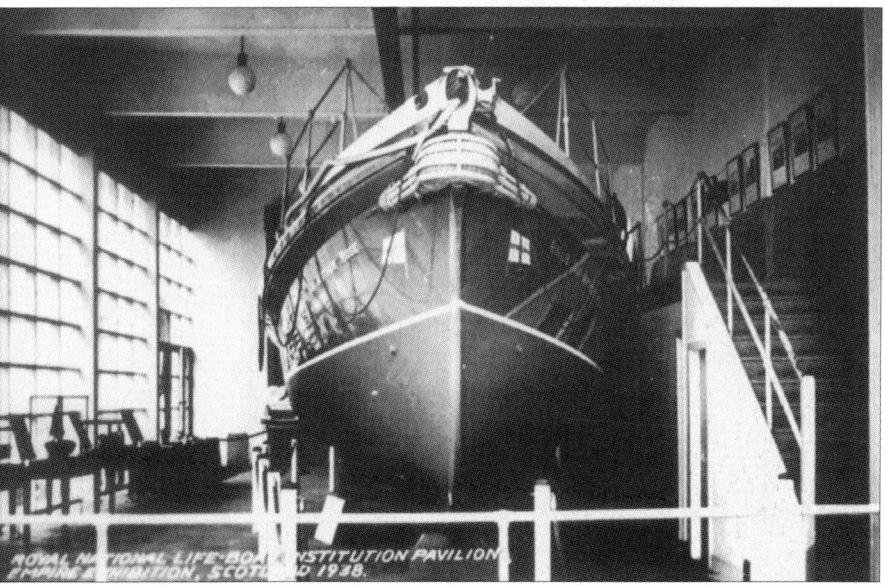

Two views of the *Sir Arthur Rose* taken at the Empire Exhibition in Glasgow in 1938
Photographs courtesy of Jeff Morris.

HOME FROM THE SEA

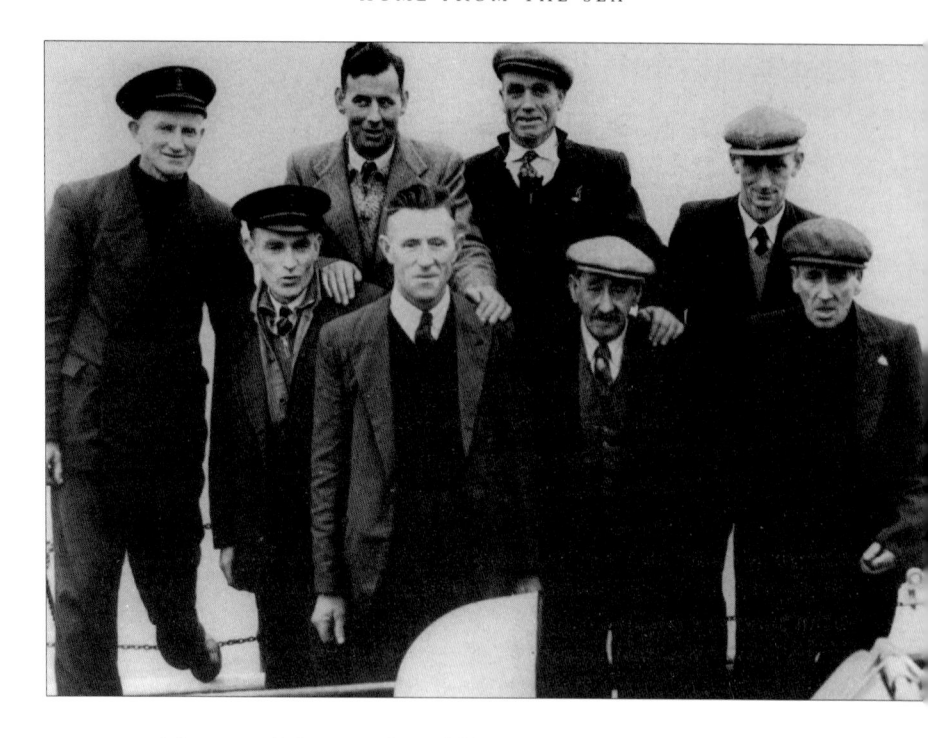

The crew of Courtmacsherry lifeboat pictured on February 16 th. 1958 Pictured at rear (l to R) John Barry, Brendan Madden, Paddy Keohane, Denis Lawton, front (L to R) William Barry, Jack Donovan, Denis Whelton, and James Whelton.
Picture courtesy of the Cork Examiner

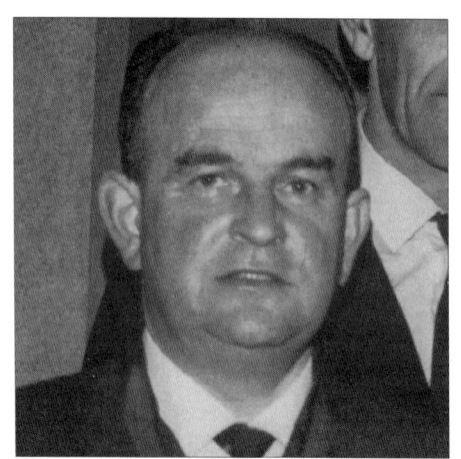

Dr. Mackillop, Hon. Sec. 1957 – 1962

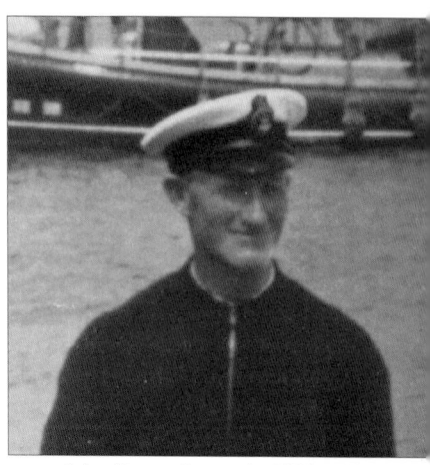

John Barry, Coxswain 1952 – 1974

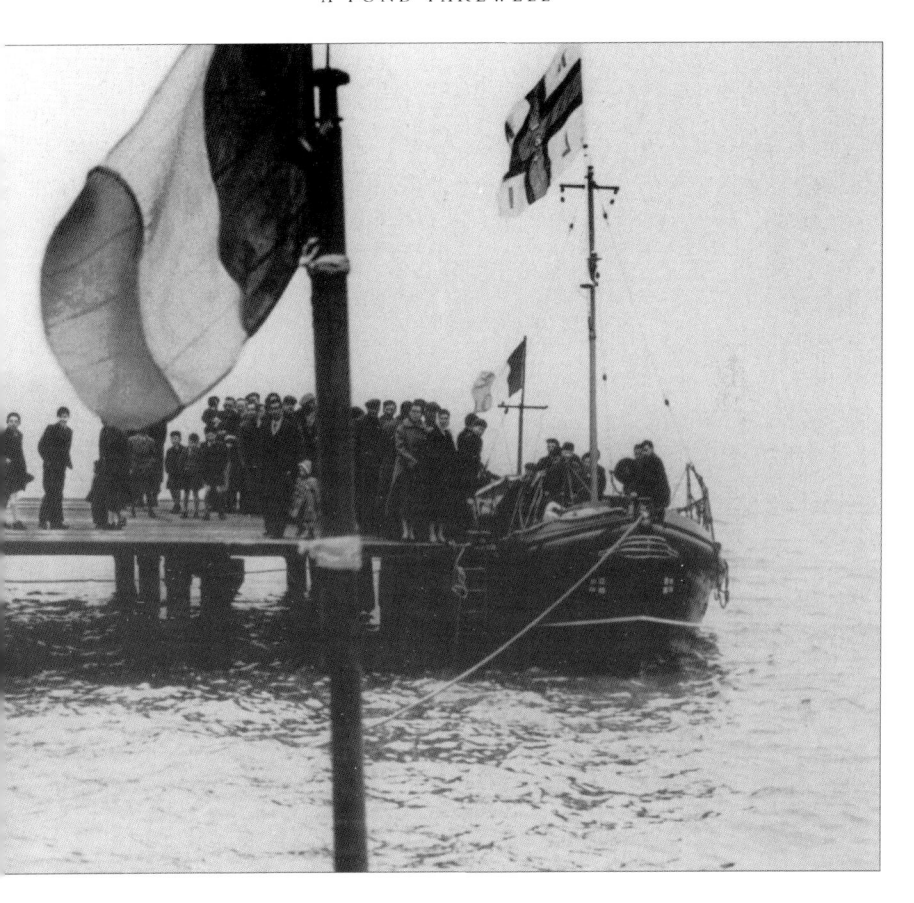

The arrival of *Sir Arthur Rose* at Courtmacsherry pier on February 16th. 1958. In the foreground is the *Sarah Ward and William David Crossweller* which had served since 1929.

Photo courtesy of the Cork Examiner.

ook place, also, in the local R.N.L.I. organisation. John Barry took over as Coxswain in 1952, a position he held for twenty two years. Johnny, as he was known locally, was eeped in the sea, having his own trawler and salmon boats as well. Dr. McKillop icceeded Frank Ruddock as Honorary Secretary in 1957.

There was a wide variety of Lifeboat services during the 1950's from small fishing oats overdue to false alarms. There was, however, a service on the 2nd. November 1955 orthy of note during 60 m.p.h. winds, probably one of the roughest seas *Sarah Ward nd William David Crossweller,* ever experienced. Shortly after 6.00 am, the *Sarah Ward nd William David Crossweller* slipped her moorings to head west for the Galley Head. he Lighthouse Keepers there received an S.O.S. from an 860 ton cargo ship, the *S.S.*

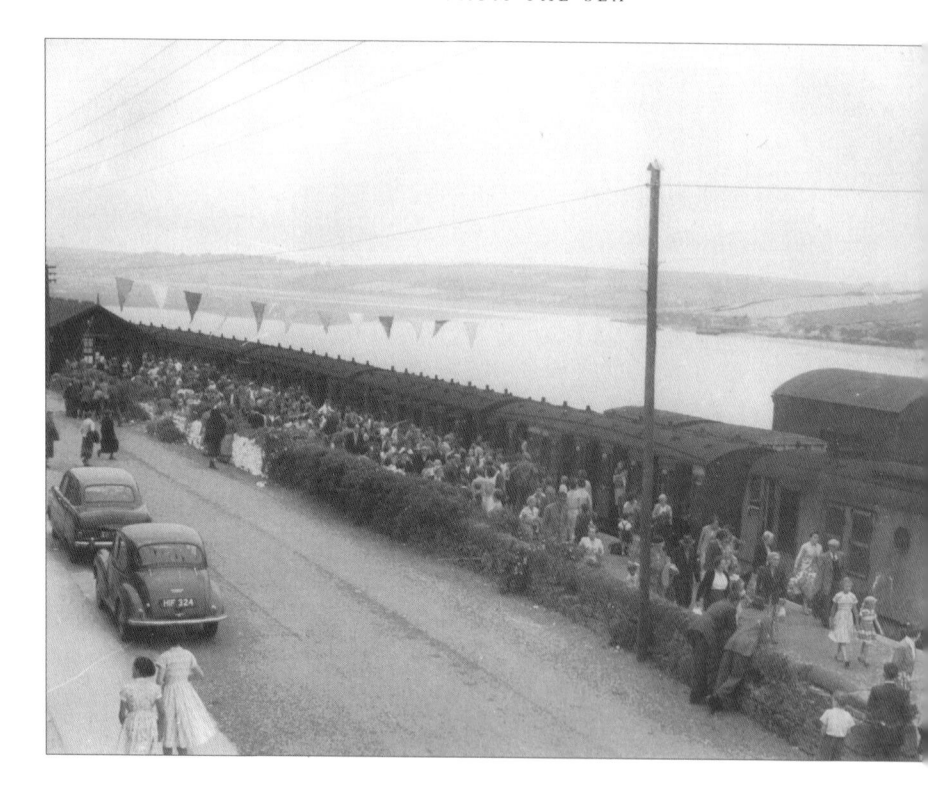

An excursion train just after arriving on Thursday August 6th. 1959 bringing a large crowd to see the annual Regatta.

Photograph courtesy of the Cork Examiner

Marioute M of London, with engine problems. Bound from Hamburg to Foynes in Co Limerick, with a load of potash, the Captain was afraid the hatches would not stand up to the battering of the mountainous seas. Ashore the storm caused widespread flooding in Clonakilty and Kinsale towns. After carrying out a search off the Galley, the Lifeboat was joined by a Shackleton Air Sea rescue plane who located the ship twelve miles south of the Galley. The Lifeboat stood by for a while until the **Marioute M** was able to head for Cork harbour under her own power.

February 1958, saw **Sarah Ward and William David Crossweller's** career in Courtmacsherry come to an end. In twenty nine years at Courtmacsherry she launched forty seven times saving sixty three lives. After leaving Courtmacsherry she served as relief Lifeboat until 1960 before being stationed at Whitehills in north east Scotland until 1961. Curiously, she is still sailing on, having been sold by the R.N.L.I. in 1961. She was converted to a pleasure boat and was last known to be based in the Channel Islands and is appropriately named **Courtmacsherry.**

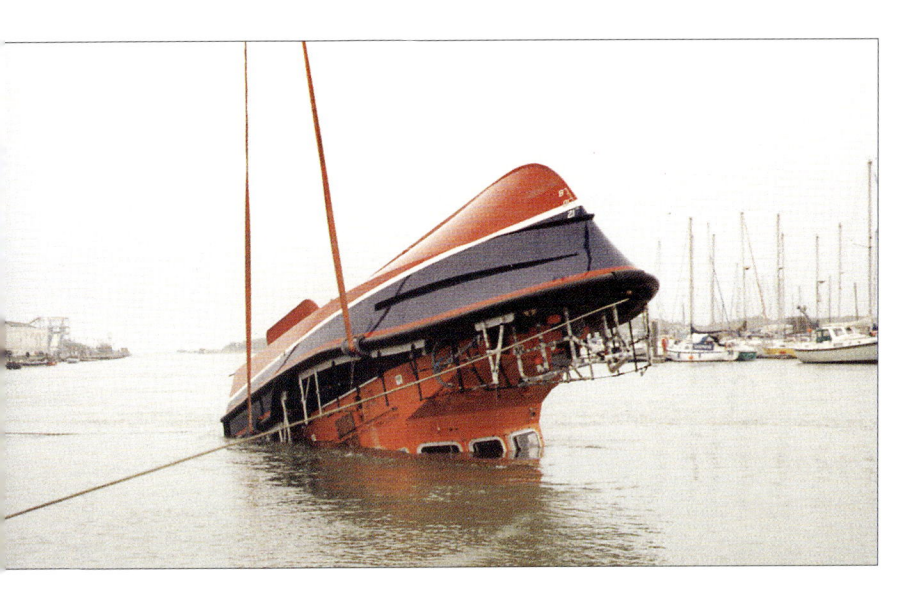

As we hope we will never see her again! ***Frederick Storey Cockburn*** undergoing her self-righting trial at Littlehampton in December 1994.

Photograph courtesy of Jim Crowley

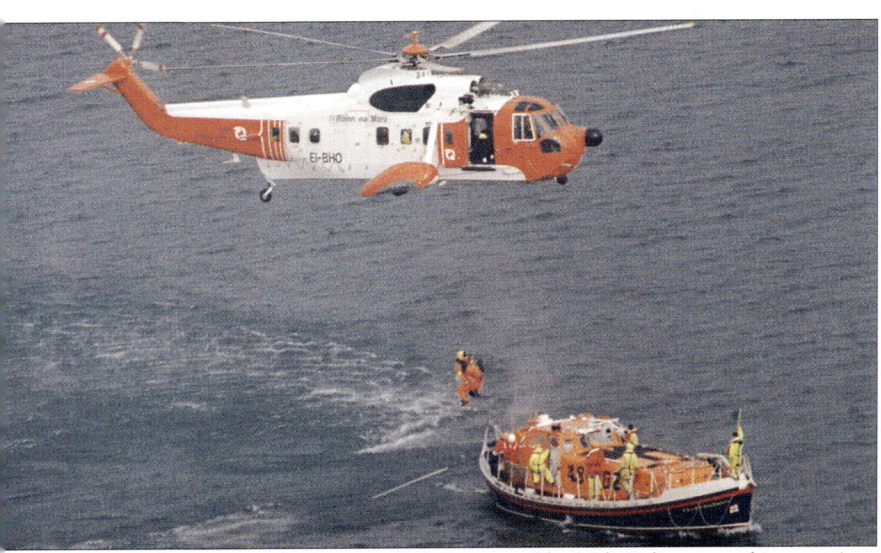

he Dept of the Marine rescue helicopter which is operated by Irish Helicopters taking part in a ombined exercise on the 20th of August 1992 at the Old Head of Kinsale with Courtmacsherry Lifeboat, ***R. Hope Roberts*** and the Old Head Cliff and Rescue Service.

Photograph courtesy of the Cork Examiner

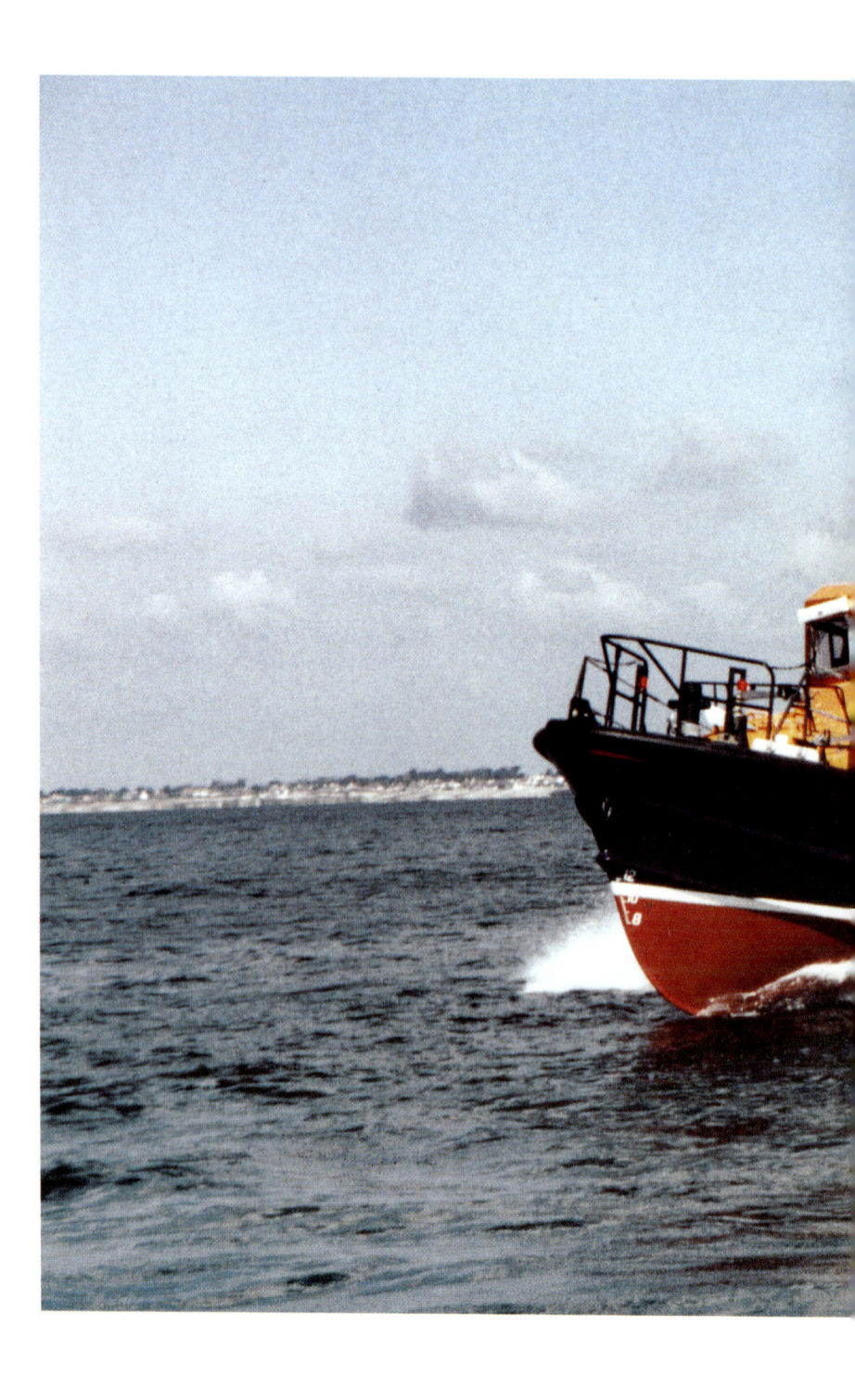

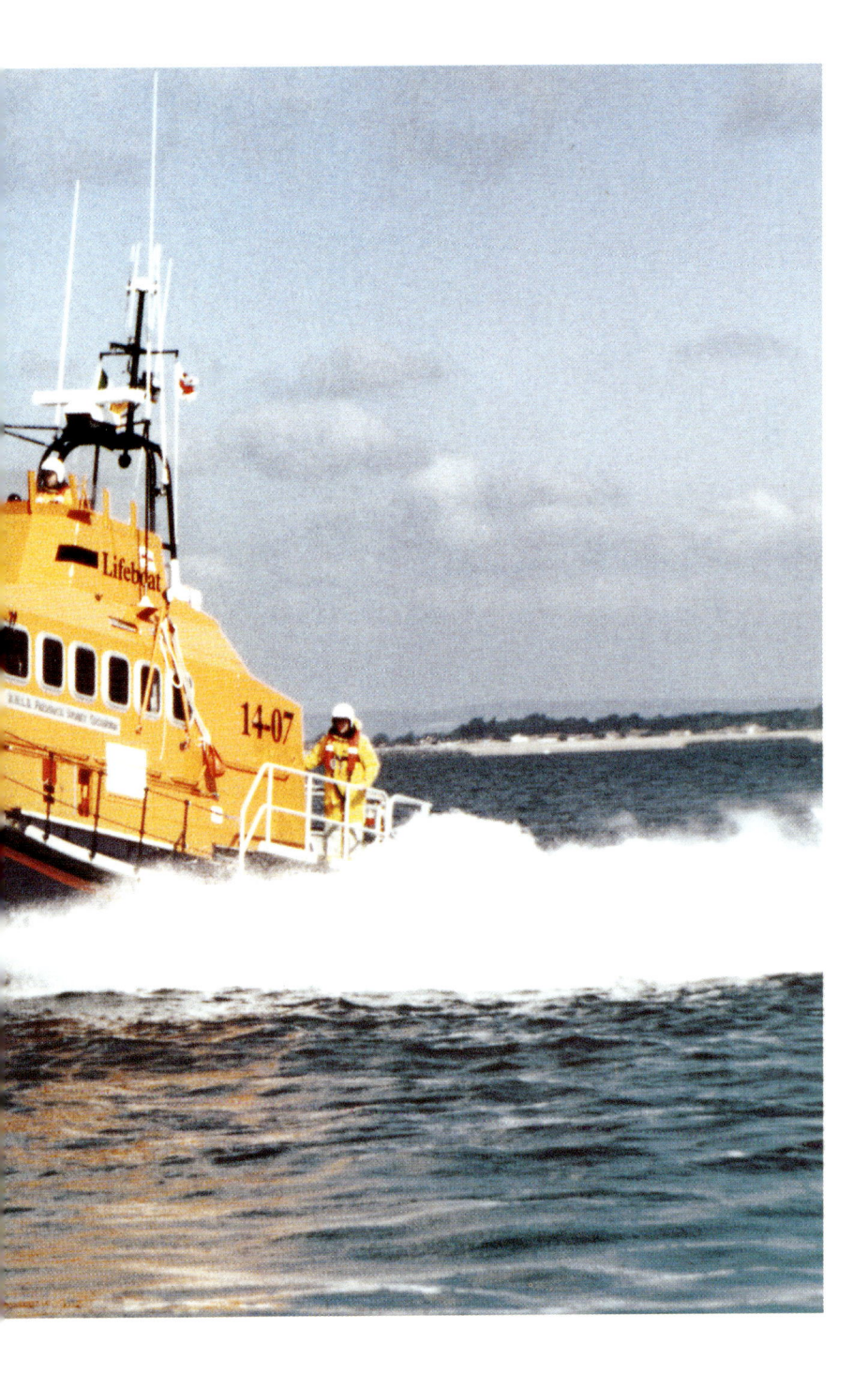

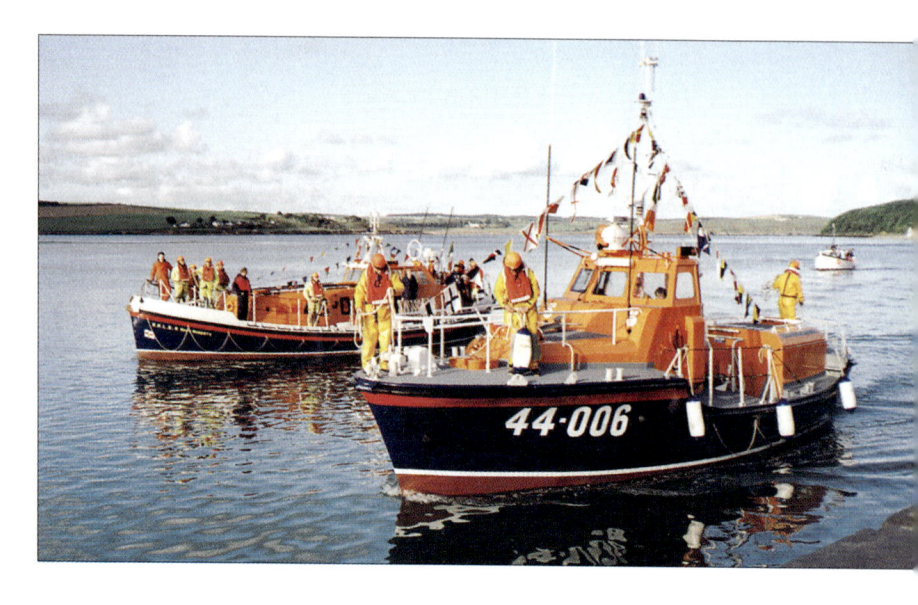

The ***Arthur and Blanche Harris*** arrives at Courtmacsherry on May 19th 1993 following her passage from Poole via Salcombe, Newlyn, Milford Haven and Dunmore East. She is being escorted by the **R. Hope Roberts**

Photograph courtesy of Vincent & Ann O'Donova

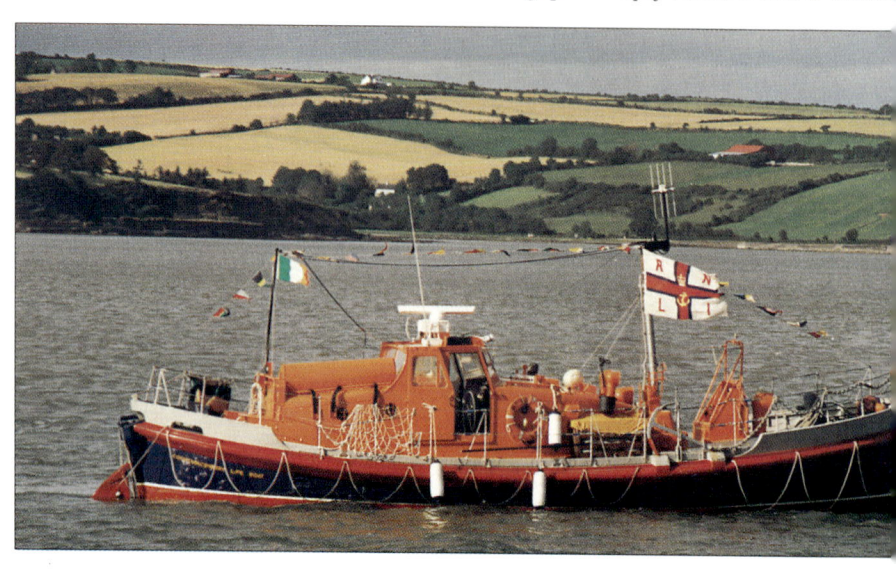

The ***Helen Wycherly*** (O.N. 959) dressed overall as she sits at her moorings in Courtmacsherry Harbour.

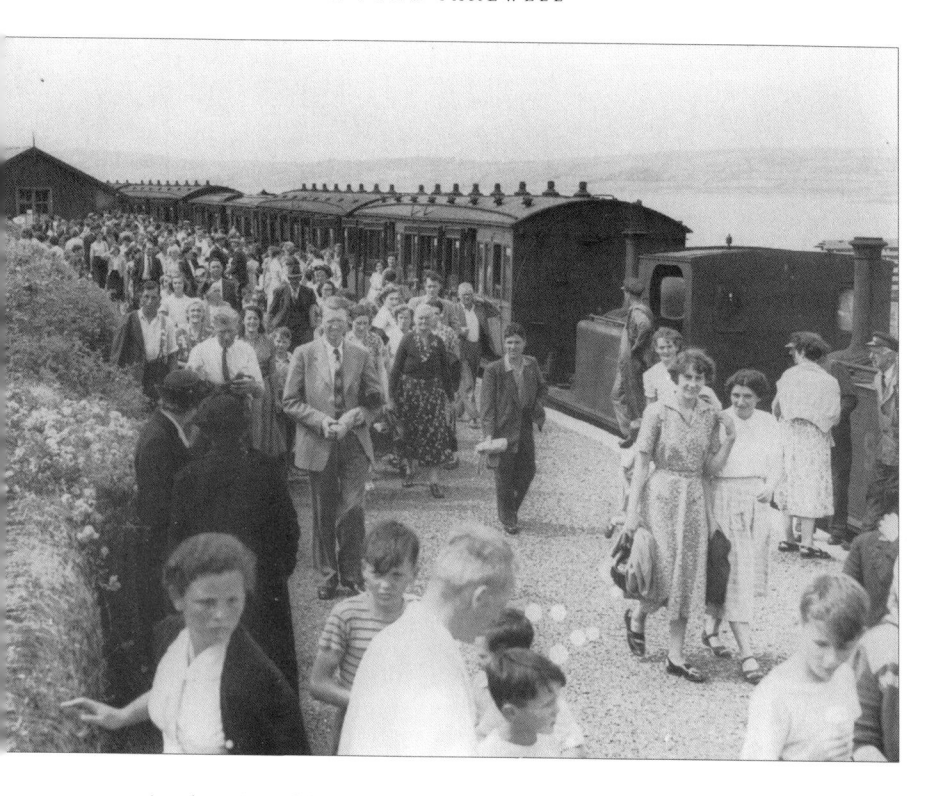

Another view of the crowd arriving by train on August 6th. 1959.
Photo courtesy of the Cork Examiner.

The arrival of **Sir Arthur Rose** (o.n. 801) on February 16th, 1958 marked a further development in Lifeboat technology. She was fitted with twin diesel 40 h.p. engines instead of petrol which had been the practice until now. The use of diesel, as well as reducing the risk of fire, also, made them more reliable and would give the Lifeboat twice the radius of her predecessor. **Sir Arthur Rose** was a 46 foot long, Watson Class, built at a cost of £8,358 by Alexander Robertson and Sons. Originally built in 1938 for Tobermory in Scotland, the boat was displayed on the R.N.L.I. pavilion at the Empire Exhibition, Glasgow 1938, prior to going into service.

She came to Courtmacsherry as a veteran of seventy one launches and ninety six lives saved between Tobermory and Mallaig. Now after a refit, she prepared for service on the coast of Cork.

Coxswain John Barry travelled to Ballycotton to join her on the last leg of the trip from the Dublin boatyard. A welcoming crowd gathered at the pier and the blessing was conducted by Rev. Fr. P. Young P.P. assisted by Rev. Fr. P. Young P.P. assisted by Rev. C. Casey, C.C. before a large crowd.

CHAPTER 12
THE END OF THE LINE
1960 – 1969

How still,
How Strangely still
The water is today.
It is not good
For water
To be so still that way.
Sea Calm by Langston Hughes 1959.

Life in Courtmacsherry in the 60's changed dramatically. The railway, which had been such a valuable asset from an economic point of view, closed in 1961.

All local and political lobbying had failed to prevent the closure, a vibrant service was gone for good. Since it's opening in 1891 it had brought thousands of tourists to the village on it's famous excursions. Sugar beet was transported to Mallow factory and sand which was landed onto the pier from the sand barges, was shovelled into wagons for onward transport to farmers inland. The little row of houses in Siberia past which the trains puffed on their journey to Timoleague, having some years previously been condemned and vacated, were now being demolished to make way for a new park. The cottages of Siberia were like an academy for Lifeboatmen, several coxswains and crewmen resided there.

It was not all decay and closures though, during this decade, a new caravan park was opened and the local Hotel changed hands and was extensively up graded. The port was busy with coasters bringing coal, fertiliser and slag for the local co-operatives. As young fellows, on our way home from school, we enjoyed going aboard and getting coins from faraway places, a collection I still have to this day.

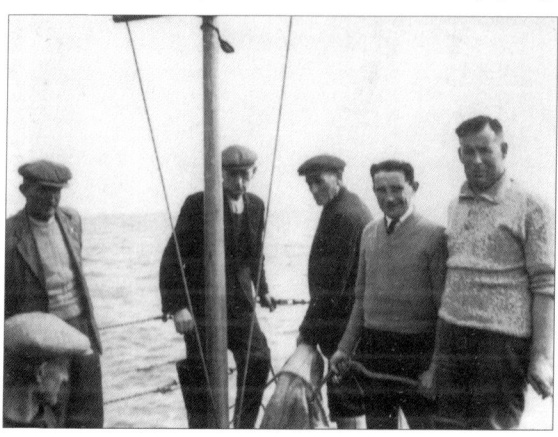

It was in 1966 that I and many more got our first glimpse of a helicopter when an Irish Air Corps helicopter landed on the pier before then proceeding to carry out an exercise with the

The crew about to "shoot" the drogue on exercise in the early 1960's
Photograph courtesy of Maureen O'Mahony

54

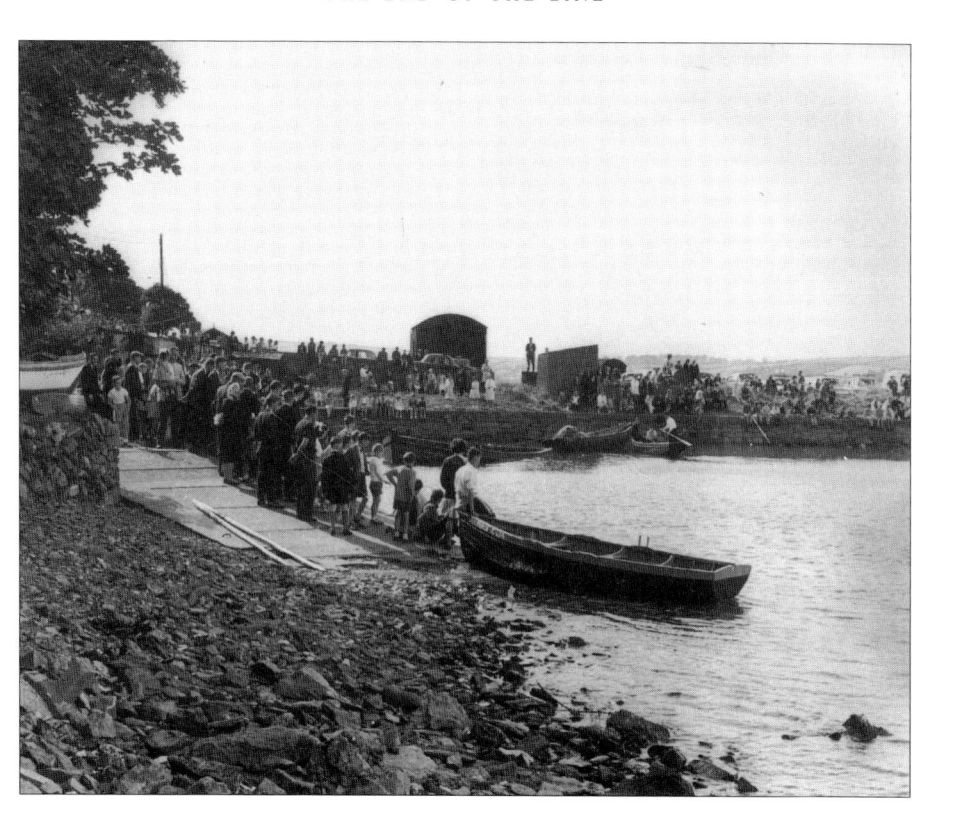

A busy scene in the dock at the pier on Thursday August 6th. 1964 as the annual regatta is in full swing. Note one of the old railway sheds in the background.

Photograph courtesy of the Cork Examiner.

Lifeboat. The end of the railway, however, brought an opportunity to improve facilities at the pier. An energetic local committee, led by retired schoolteacher, Padraig O'Cochláin, acquired a portion of the former railway station property, in 1966, and constructed a new slipway and Angling Centre, which are still in use.

The *Sir Arthur Rose* was continuing her proud tradition and, in the period 1960 - 1969, launched no fewer than 21 times. On the night of February 18th/19th, 1969 *Sir Arthur Rose* went to the aid of a French trawler *Obeline* broken down and drifting only about half a mile south of Old Head in a force ten gale with a very rough sea. Due to conditions, at the bar at Courtmacsherry, the Lifeboat decided to remain at sea for the night and stood by the *Obeline* while another French vessel had her in tow. The Lifeboat returned to Courtmacsherry at 10.00am, the casualty having been towed to Kinsale. One of the crew on that night was Jim Crowley who is now one of the Deputy Launching Authorities.

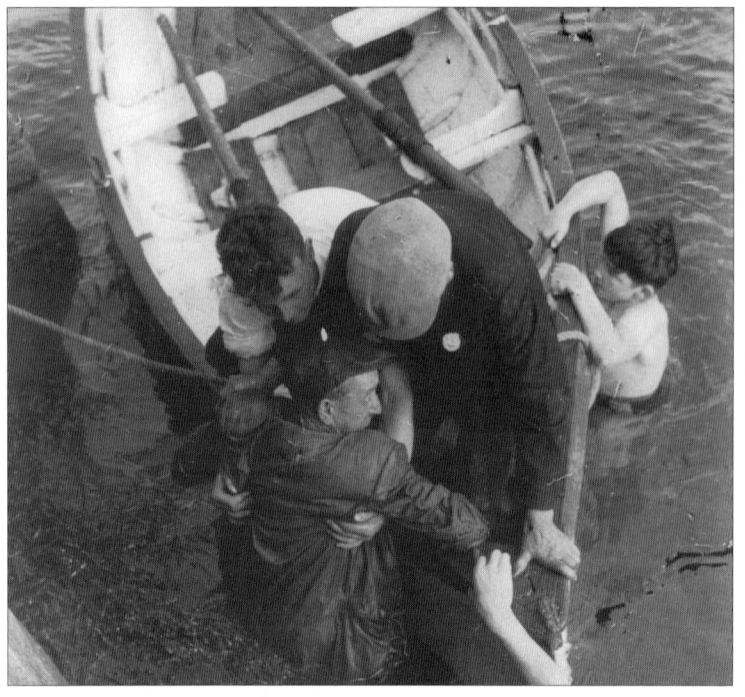

A lucky escape for former Lifeboat crewman, John Whelton who fell into the water while while "greasing" the pole during the Regatta on the 6th. of August. He is being helped up by his brother Denis also a former Lifeboatman. Note the Lifeboat day badge on Denis's lapel!

Photograph courtesy of the Cork Examiner.

In August 1969, another big improvement for the lifeboat station was about to take place. The **Helen Wycherley** was to replace *Sir Arthur Rose*. The new boat was built by Groves and Guttridge on the Isle of Wight in 1961 at a cost of £35,500. The money was provided out of a legacy of Mr. Harry Wycherley of Rochdale, a gift from Miss Jane Robb and the R.N.L.I.'s own funds. It was named after Mr. Wycherley's wife. This Lifeboat, weighing 22 ton and 46 foot 9 inches long, was wooden hulled with watertight compartments to assist buoyancy. She was propelled by two 60 h.p. diesel engines which would give her a speed of nearly 9 knots. The most dramatic improvement though, was the enclosed wheelhouse amidships. At last, this would give the Coxswain and crew some bit of comfort from the elements outside.

The Lifeboat underwent a major refit at Crosshaven Boatyard under the direction of Noble Ruddock, District Engineer, after her arrival from Whitehills in Scotland, where she had served since she was first built. The Lifeboat arrived in Courtmacsherry on Saturday August 23rd having left Crosshaven on trials via Baltimore and the Fastnet. Many small boats, bedecked with flags, met the **Helen Wycherley** at the mouth of the harbour to welcome her in. I was lucky enough to have got a spin out on a small boat owned by Patrick Fleming, owner of the Anchor Bar. Arriving at the pier, a large crowd were present to greet her.

Are-dedication ceremony then took place with Very Rev. P. Fullam P.P. performing

THE END OF THE LINE

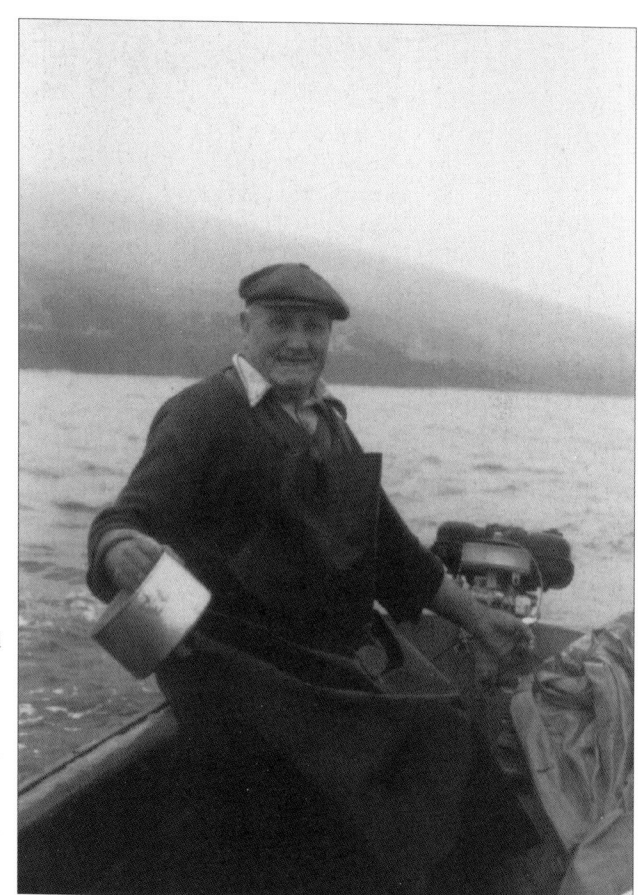

Paddy Keohane who served on the lifeboat crew for many years and was coxswain from 1974 until his retirement in 1977.
He is pictured here out in his own boat tending to his lobster pots.

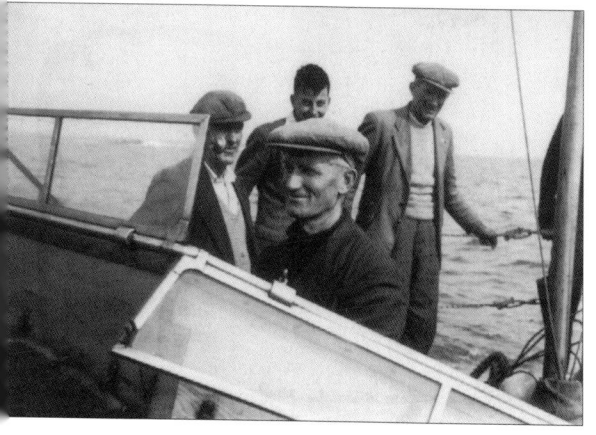

Coxswain John Barry and crew on exercise with ***Sir Arthur Rose*** Lifeboat probably in the early 1960's

Photograph courtesy of Maureen O' Mahony..

the blessing assisted by Rev James Coombes.C.C.

In attendance for the ceremony were Mr. G. E. Walton, R.N.L.I. District Inspector, and Mr. Noble Ruddock, a native of Courtmacsherry the R.N.L.I. District Engineer for Ireland. The crew of the new Lifeboat were:

> *John Barry Coxswain*
> *Brendan Madden Mechanic*
> *Jack Madden*
> *Denis Lawton*
> *Paddy Keohane 2nd. Coxswain*
> *Jim Crowley*
> *Seamus Barry*

The arrival and blessing of the *Helen Wycherley* was tinged with a little sadness as her sister ship, the *T.G.B,* stationed at Longhope in Scotland, had capsized on 17th March during a service to a Liberian Ship. All eight of the Lifeboat crew were drowned when the *T.G.B.* remained upside down having capsized in a force nine gale. Many Lifeboats, at the time, were not self righting, as they were considered too unstable, and crews did

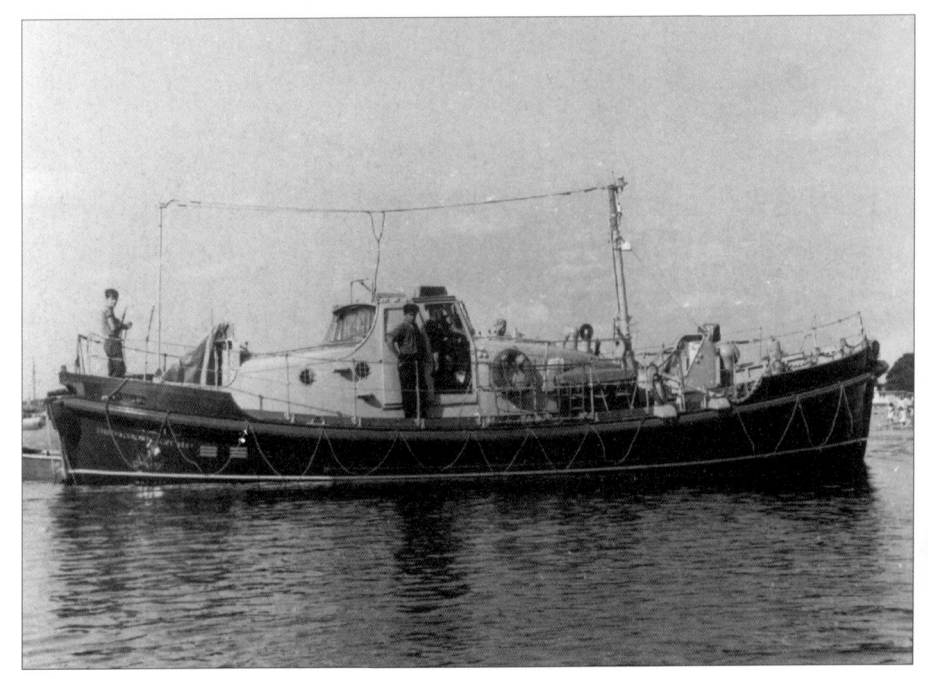

The *Helen Wycherley* at Crosshaven following her refit before coming to Courtmacsherry.
Photograph courtesy of the Cork Examiner.

THE END OF THE LINE

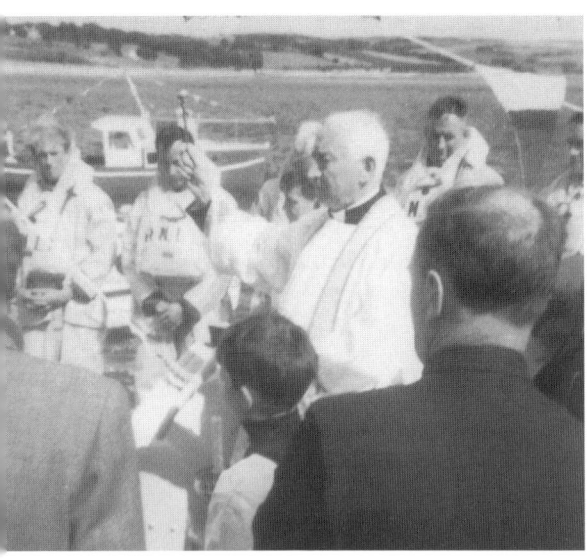

The blessing and re-dedication of the **Helen Wycherley** on Saturday the 23rd. of August 1969.
Photograph courtesy of the Cork Examiner.

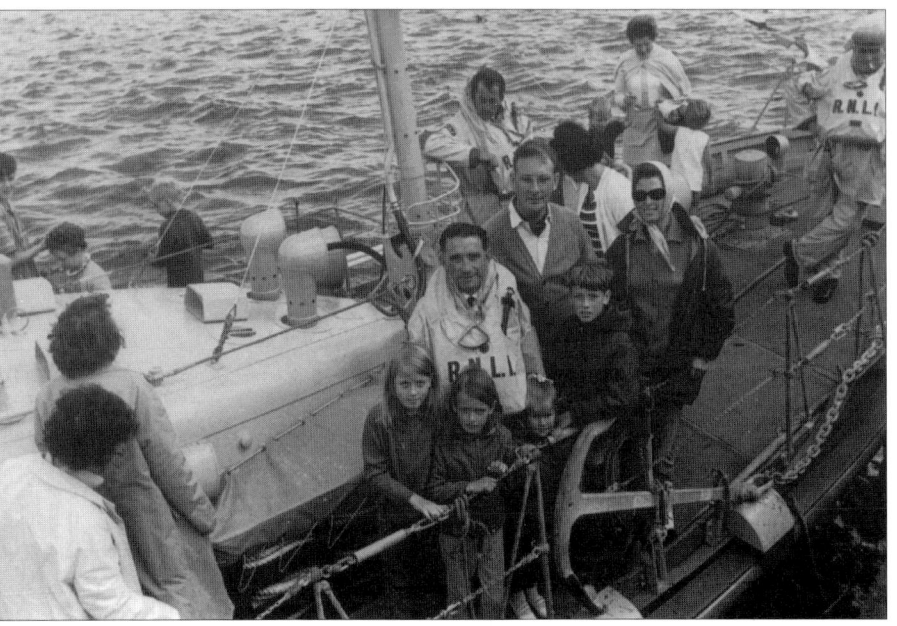

Visitors are being shown around the new lifeboat while Second coxswain Paddy Keohane enjoys a quiet smoke!
Photograph courtesy of the Cork Examiner.

not like them. However, several other disasters, in the mid 50's, had already resulted in a major review of self righting versus non-self righting. New boats of the Oakley Class, introduced in 1958, were inherently self-righting. The R.N.L.I. put in place a conversion programme to fit the Watson Class Lifeboats with an air bag that would inflate upon capsize and automatically right the boat. (The **Helen Wycherley** was modified in 1974).

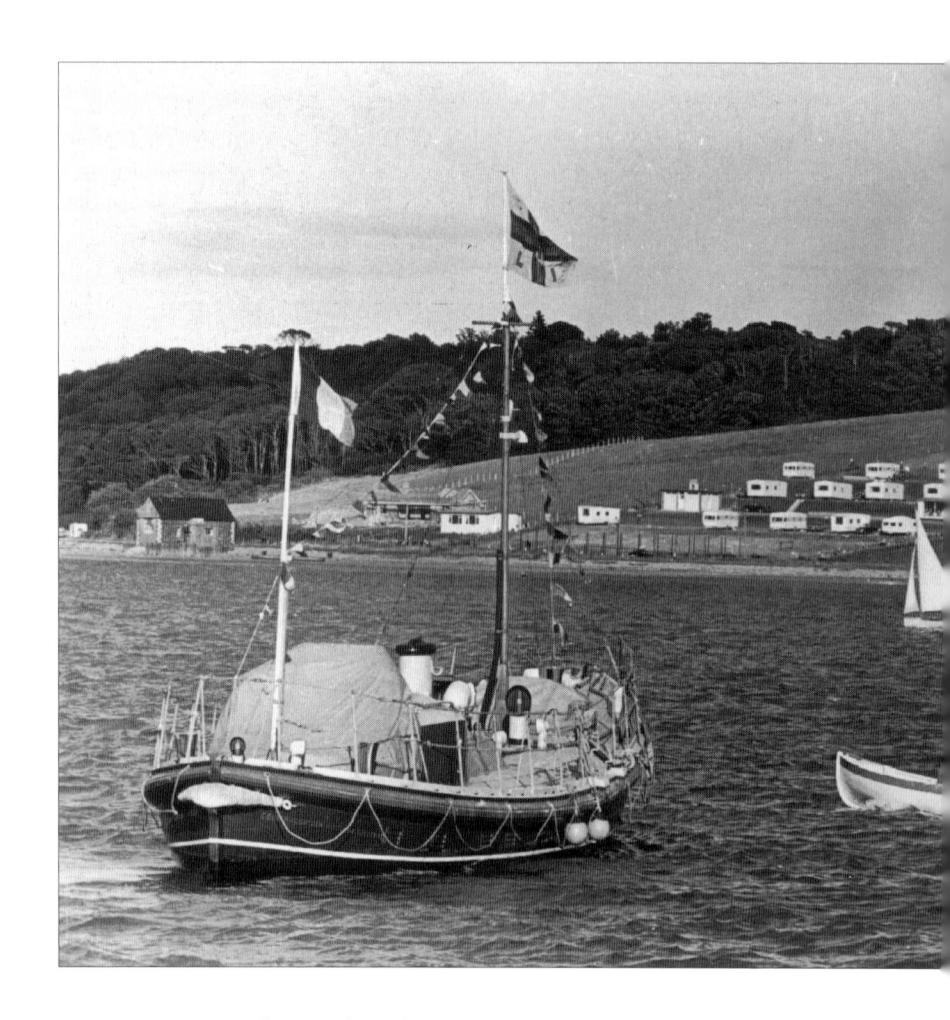

Sir Arthur Rose lies at her moorings on Thursday August 4th 1966, the day of the Annual Regatta.

Photograph courtesy of the Cork Examiner

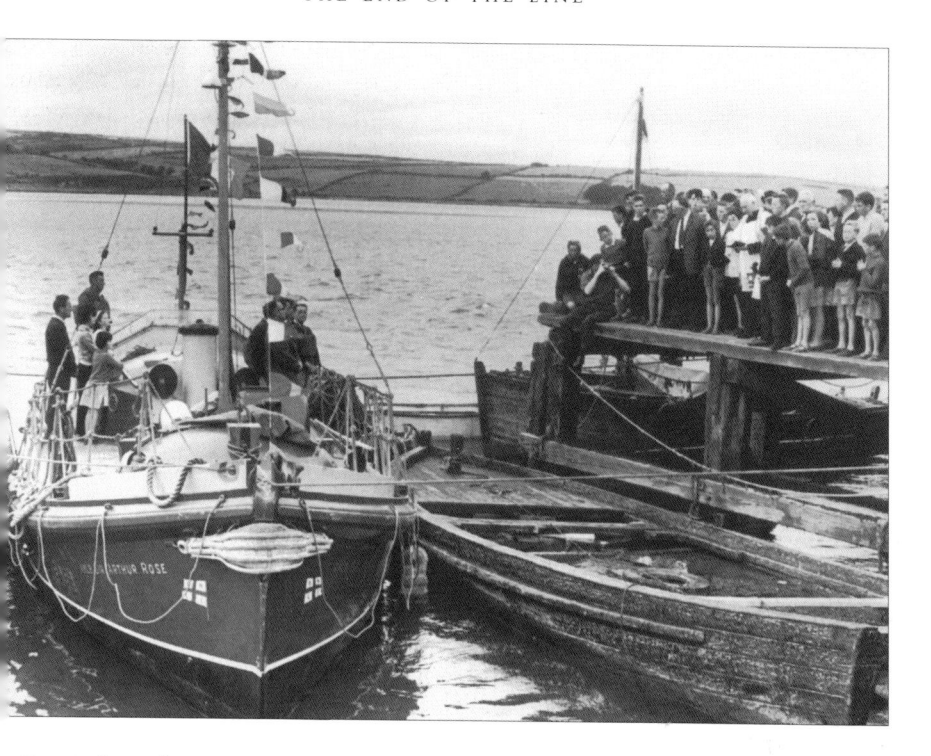

Rev. Father Fullam Parish Priest of Barryroe conducting the blessing of the new slipway and angling centre on Saturday evening July 30th 1966.
Sir Arthur Rose is alongside the large jetty for the occasion.

Photograph courtesy of the Cork Examiner.

CHAPTER 13
THE FASTNET RACE
1970 – 1979

> Obscurest night involved the sky,
> The Atlantic billows roared,
> When such a destined wretch as I,
> Washed headlong from on board,
> Of friends, of hope, of all bereft,
> His floating home for ever left.
>
> *From The Castaway by William Cowper 1803.*

THE ***Helen Wycherley*** had by now settled into the local landscape and the early year consisted of the usual selection of rescues, fishing boats broken down or overdue.

The village enjoyed a boom time in May 1970 when, due to a cement strike, a large number of coasters came to the pier with cement from abroad.

Ships were unloaded twenty four hours a day and lorries, from all over Ireland, queued on the road waiting for their precious load. The local pubs did a roaring trade as thirsty dockers had to be supplied, on board, with suitable refreshment.

The frenzy was so great that any bag falling off the hastily loaded lorries would not be reclaimed except by another group of entrepreneurs who would sweep it up and bag it for resale locally. It was not unusual to have three boats waiting at the pier to be unloaded and one or two more waiting in the Bay for their turn.

Several of the Lifeboat crew were employed and, for many, real money was earned for the very first time.

1976 saw the untimely death of Mr John O'Dwyer N.T., who had been Honorary Secretary since 1962. He was succeeded by Mr. Desmond Bateman, who up to that time, had been Deputy Launching Authority. Sea angling had, by now, become a thriving summer attraction and visitors came from all over Europe to fish for blue shark or ground fishing for the plentiful conger, ling and pollack. Up to eight boats would be required some weekends to cater for the visitors. It was to one such boat, in August, 1977, that I got my real initiation

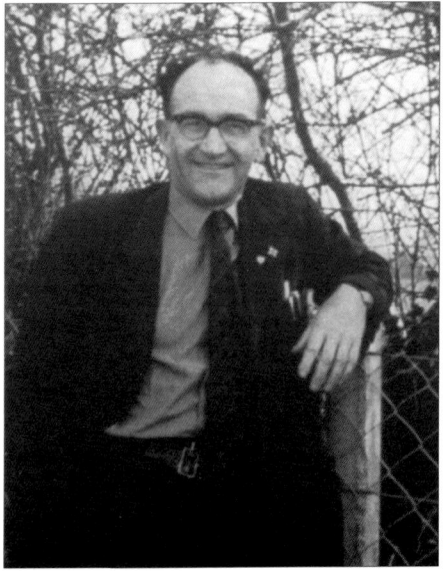

John o' Dwyer N.T. Hon. Sec. of Courtmacsherry lifeboat from 1962 until 1976.

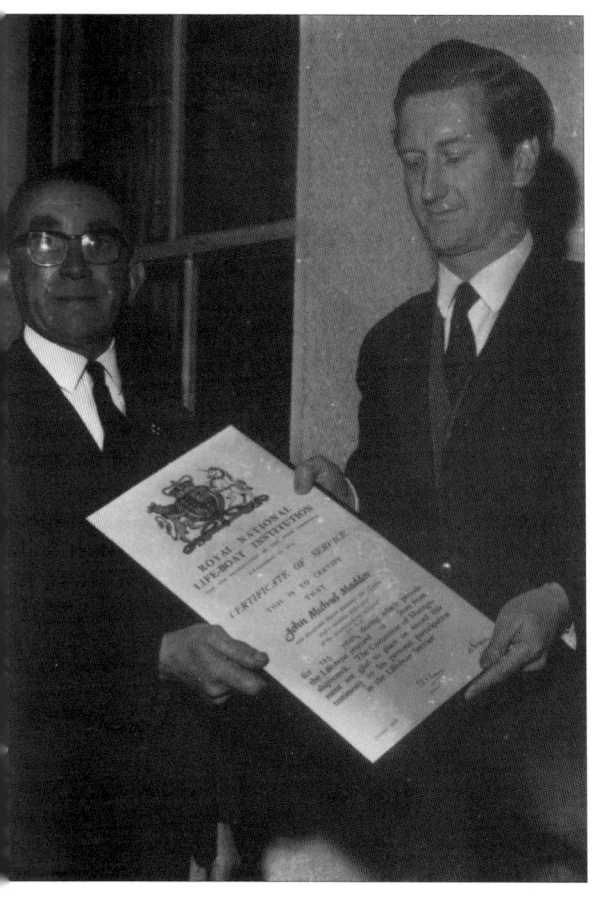

into Lifeboat work.

A local angling boat was broken down with seven persons on board off the Old Head of Kinsale. As *Joseph Hiram Chadwick*, which was on relief duty, approached the **St. Anthony**, I could see the terrified faces of a few small children in their mothers arms as they wallowed about in the choppy sea. Soon we would have them in tow and take them to calm waters and the safety of Courtmacsherry harbour. It is at that moment the bug of Lifeboating hits you and, for which, to my knowledge, there is no known cure!

August 14th 1979, however, was to be far more that a simple trip across the bay to tow home a broken down boat. The shrill ring of the telephone at 1.40am brought the Honorary Secretary, Des Bateman, quickly into action. Valentia Radio were seeking an immediate launch of the Lifeboat to go to the assistance of the yacht **Wild Goose** in difficulties some 27 miles south of the Old Head of Kinsale.

Jack Madden being presented with a Vellum Certificate on his retirement from the crew of Courtmacsherry Lifeboat in 1973 by Lt. Commander Brian Miles the then district inspector of the RNLI. in Ireland.
Jack had served on the crew for a total of 15 years, 8 of those as assistant mechanic.
Photograph courtesy of Michael Minihane.

Des Bateman had barely **received the message when the telephone went dead, the telephone exchange in Bandon having been struck by lightning.**

The Honorary Secretary was left with no option but to drive the three miles from his house near Timoleague to round up the crew. The loud bang of the maroons rang out at 2.20am and *Sir Samuel Kelly*, which was on relief duty at Courtmacsherry, slipped her moorings at 2.40am.

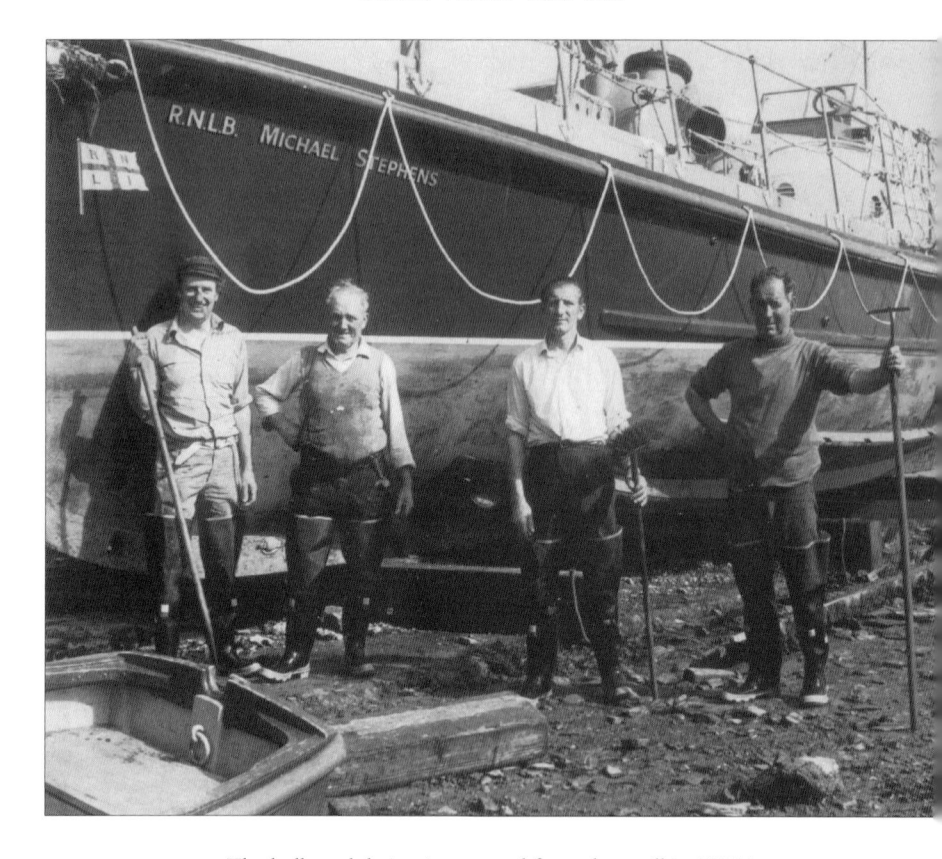

The hull scrub being interrupted for a photocall in 1974 !
This was taken while the **Michael Stephens** was on relief duty at Courtmacsherry.
The station boat, **Helen Wycherley,** was away for a major refit.
Pictured (L to R) Sam Mearns, Paddy Keohane, Tom Mulcahy and Brendan Madden.

Coxswain Sam Mearns was in control and after clearing the mouth of the harbour course was set for the yacht's position. By 3.20am, however, Ballycotton Lifeboat had also launched to go to the aid of **Wild Goose** so, having been requested by the Naval Vessel **L.E. Deirdre** to divert to a position 30 miles south of the Galley Head, Courtmacsherry Lifeboat went to the aid of the yacht **Pepsi** which was also in difficulties. Coxswain Mearns altered course which then brought **Sir Samuel Kelly** heading directly into mountainous seas with the wind blowing up to force 10 making conditions almost unbearable. At 8.40am, the Lifeboat was at the **Pepsi**'s reported position but no trace of her was found. A search was therefore initiated. From that time until 10.00am, two more yachts were located but were in full control and not in need of any assistance.

At 10.00a.m. the British yacht **Casse Tete 5** reported, on VHF radio, that she had lost

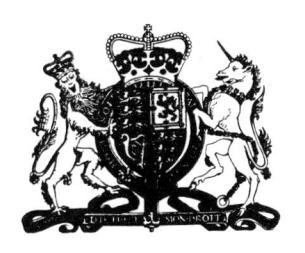

AT A MEETING OF
THE COMMITTEE OF MANAGEMENT
OF THE
ROYAL NATIONAL LIFE-BOAT INSTITUTION
FOR THE PRESERVATION OF LIFE FROM
SHIPWRECK
HELD ON THE ELEVENTH DAY OF DECEMBER, 1974,
THE FOLLOWING MINUTE WAS ORDERED TO BE
RECORDED ON THE BOOKS OF THE INSTITUTION

THAT THE INSTITUTION GRATEFULLY
RECOGNISES THE SERVICES OF THE
COURTMACSHERRY HARBOUR, CO. CORK LIFE-BOAT STATION
ESTABLISHED IN 1825

IN THE GREAT CAUSE OF LIFE-SAVING FROM
SHIPWRECK AND ON THE OCCASION OF THE
150TH ANNIVERSARY OF THE
STATION'S ESTABLISHMENT,
DESIRES TO PLACE ON RECORD ITS
APPRECIATION OF THE VOLUNTARY WORK
OF THE OFFICERS AND COMMITTEE AND
OF THE DEVOTION AND COURAGE
OF THE LIFE-BOAT CREWS
WHO HAVE NEVER FAILED TO MAINTAIN THE
HIGH TRADITIONS OF THE LIFE-BOAT SERVICE

F.R.H. S_____
CHAIRMAN

PRESIDENT

DIRECTOR & SECRETARY

The Vellum presented to Courtmacsherry Lifeboat Station in September 1975 to commemorate the 150 th. anniversary of the Station's establishment.

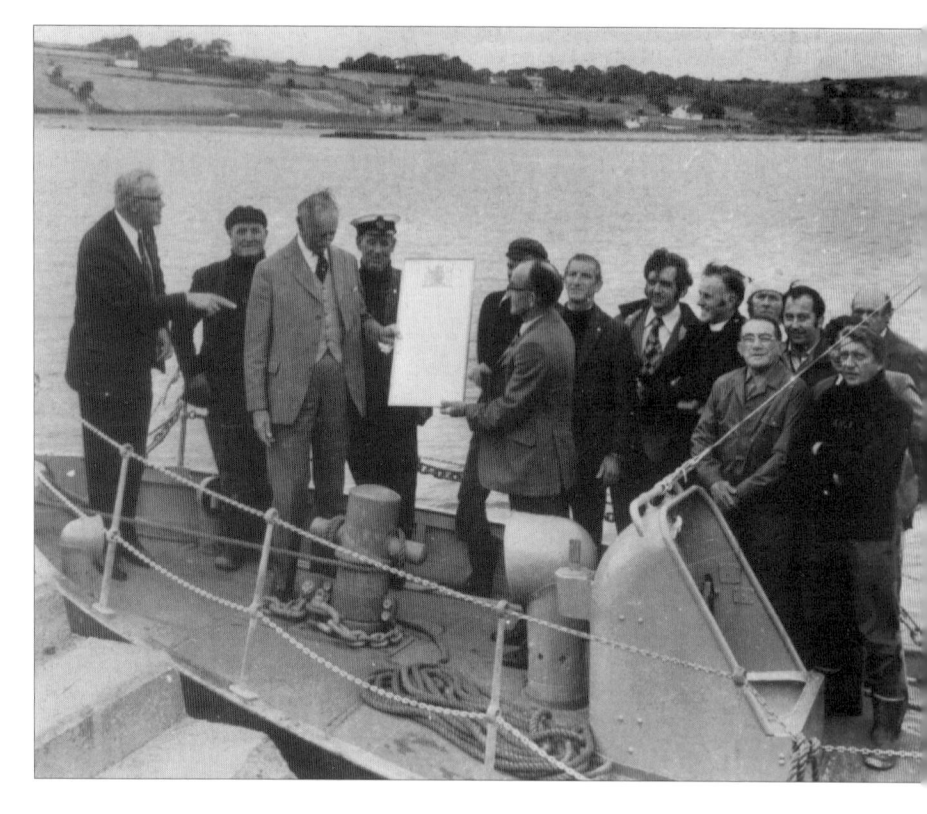

The presentation of the 150 th anniversary vellum to John o'Dwyer Hon. Sec. on board the lifeboat in September 1975.

Photograph courtesy of Michael Minihane.

her rudder 26 miles south of the Galley Head. This meant that **Sir Samuel Kelly** was not far from this position. In the absence of communication with **Pepsi** or more definite information as to her whereabouts, a decision was taken to head for **Casse Tete 5**.

The **Casse Tete 5**, like all the other yachts of that fateful night, were taking part in the bi-annual Fastnet race. This race is a mecca for many yachtsmen. 303 yachts began the race on August 11th from Cowes on the Isle of Wight. The race would take them on a 605 mile course west around Lands End and then north-west around the famous Fastnet Rock off Baltimore, which gives the race its name, before returning around Lands End and eastwards to the finish at Plymouth. The fury of the gale that decimated the race seemed to take everyone by surprise. A low pressure area had moved eastwards quickly across the Atlantic from America, where it had caused severe damage on August 9th. Winds of up to force 8 had been forecast for the evening of August 13th but, to many yachts, this did not cause undue anxiety. Soon, however, the wind strength increased to

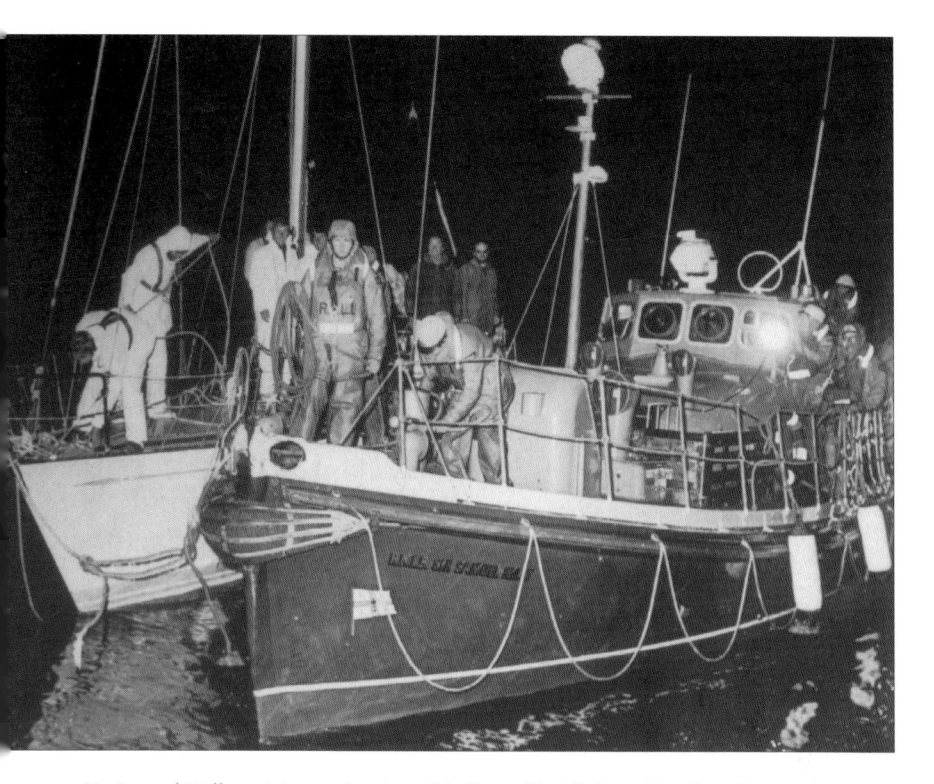

Sir Samuel Kelly arriving at the pier with *Casse Tete V* alongside after a long and difficult service on the 15th. of August 1979.

Photograph courtesy of Michael Minihane.

force 10 and the difference between force 8 and force 10 is immense. Many yachts were rolled over causing severe damage. Crews took to liferafts but these were overwhelmed or torn apart by the maelstrom.

Fifteen yachtsmen in total lost their lives. Many more were saved in the huge rescue operation which included the use of five Lifeboats on the Irish Coast, nine Lifeboats on the English coast, rescue helicopters, fixed wing aircraft, naval ships, fishing vessels and other craft. The ten yachtsmen aboard **Casse Tete 5** were amongst the lucky ones. *Sir Samuel Kelly* located them at 11.30am. and soon had a tow passed. This was extremely difficult due to the violent motion of both boats caused by up to 40 feet high waves. At 11.45am the long tow towards Courtmacsherry commenced. A speed of only a little over 2 knots was possible due to the conditions and it was midnight that night before *Sir Samuel Kelly*, with the **Casse Tete 5** in tow reached Courtmacsherry and received a fantastic welcome at Courtmacsherry Pier. A reserve crew was waiting to refuel the Lifeboat and take her to sea again, if necessary, while the crew of both Lifeboat and the

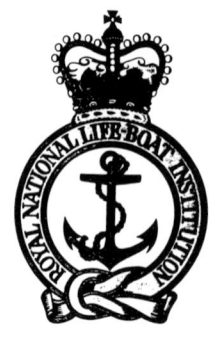

At a meeting of the Committee of Management of the
ROYAL NATIONAL LIFE-BOAT INSTITUTION
held on the 23rd January, 1980, it was resolved to award this special certificate to the Coxswain and Crew of the life-boat
"SIR SAMUEL KELLY"
ON TEMPORARY DUTY AT COURTMACSHERRY

COXSWAIN
S. Mearns

ACTING SECOND COXSWAIN
D. O'Mahony

ACTING MECHANIC
M. Gannon

EMERGENCY MECHANIC
H. Oulton

CREW MEMBERS
A. Dorman, T. Mulcahy, P. McCarthy & C. McCarthy

in recognition of the services carried out by them on the 14th August, 1979 when the yachts "Wild Goose," "Pepsi" and "Casse Tête V," competing in the Fastnet Race, were in difficulties in a west-north-westerly storm and heavy seas. The life-boat was at sea for 21½ hours and carried out a search for two of the yachts and saved the yacht "Casse Tête V" and her crew of ten.

CHAIRMAN

The Special Certificate of Thanks awarded to the Coxswain and crew of Courtmacsherry Lifeboat following the service on the night of August 15th. 1979.

yacht were treated to a welcome hot meal.

The Lifeboat, and her crew, had been at sea a total of twenty two and a half hours, which is one of the longest services in the station's proud history. A certificate of thanks was presented to the station for their outstanding determination on that difficulty day.

The crew were:-

Sam Mearns	*Coxswain*
Dermot O'Mahony	*2nd. Coxswain*
Mark Gannon	*Mechanic*
Harold Oulton	
Tony Dorman	
Tom Mulcahy	
P. J. McCarthy	
Cal McCarthy	

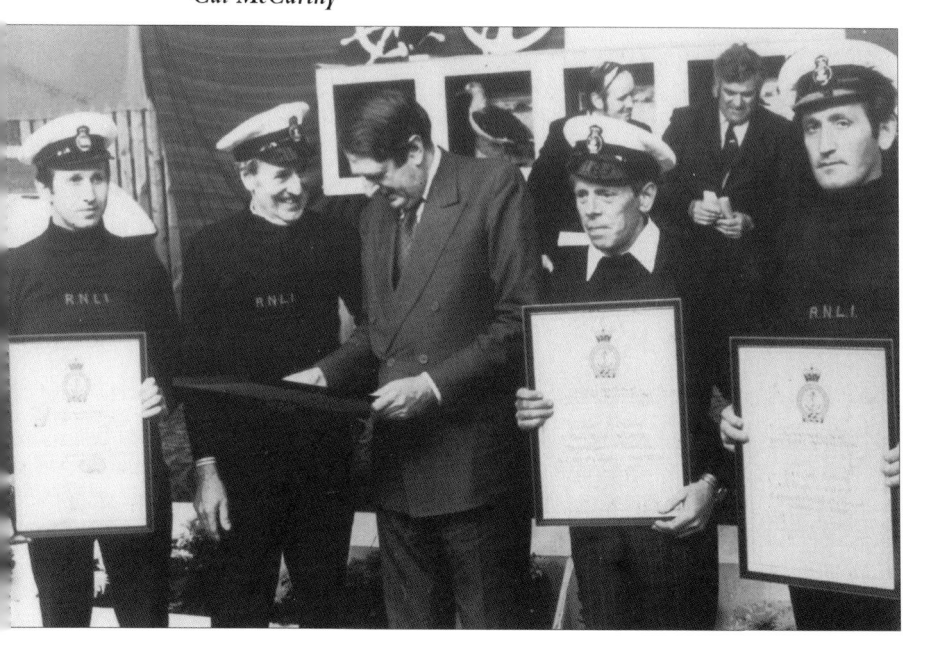

This group are pictured at the presentation of a Framed Certificate of Thanks to each of the south coast Lifeboat coxswains on behalf of their Stations for their various services on the night of the Fastnet race August 15th. 1979.

The presentation took place at the Cork boat show February 1980.
Pictured (L to R) John Walsh of Dunmore East, Sam Mearns Courtmacsherry , The Duke of Atholl, Chairman of the RNLI,
Christy Collins Baltimore and Tom Mc.Leod Ballycotton.

CHAPTER 14
CROSSING THE BAR
1980 – 1989

Sunset and evening star,
And one clear call for me!
And may there be no moaning of the bar,
When I put out to sea,

But such a tide as moving seems asleep,
Too full for sound and foam,
When that which drew out from the boundless deep
Turns home again.

Twilight and evening bell,
And after that the dark!
And may there be no sadness of farewell,
When I embark;

For tho' from out our bourne of time and place
The flood may bear me far,
I hope to see my Pilot face to face
When I have crost the bar.

Tennyson(1889

Never did any harbour exist that can conceal the true state of wind and tide out at sea as Courtmacsherry. Nestling at the base of a hill, it is sheltered from all southerly wind which can have the waters of the harbour looking serene while a full gale rages outside. So it was on Saturday afternoon December 19th, 1981. When the maroon was fired at approximately 2.00pm, I was working in a friends house at the end of the village completing an electrical job. I had to run most of the way to the boathouse as my wife had gone shopping and taken the car. As I ran, puffing, to the boathouse, I wondered what the call might be.

A Dutchman, who ran a small guesthouse and angling business, was expected, having left Holland a few days previously with a new angling boat for the forthcoming season Arriving at the boathouse I enquired from the Coxswain, Brendan Madden, as to the nature of the emergency. He told me that a boat was seen capsizing near Barry's Point. I was working and living in Cork City, at that time, so I waited until the regulars got their gear on. Then my turn came as Brendan counted out his crew, he had room for one more *"Put on your gear Micheál"* Brendan shouted and I sprung into action pulling up the

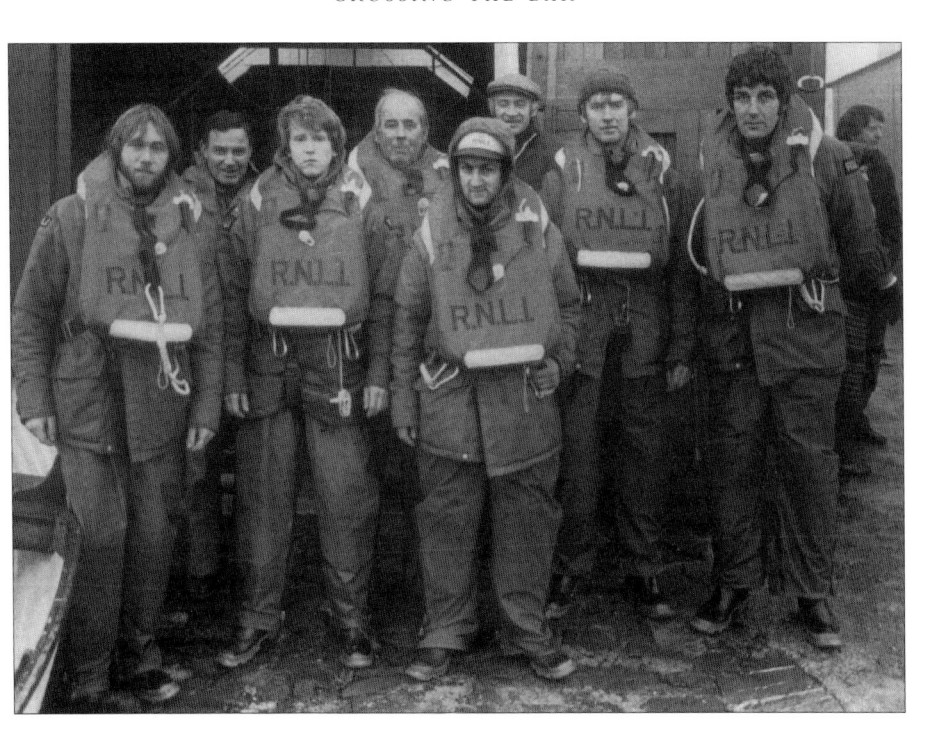

The crew of the **Helen Wycherley** pictured on Sunday morning December 20th. 1981.
(l to R) Mark Gannon, Nick Byrne, Niall O' Sullivan, Coxswain/ Mechanic
Brendan Madden, Cally McCarthy, and a weary Mícheál Hurley!
In the background is the Hon. Sec. Des Bateman, missing from the photograph is Tom Mulcahy.
Photograph courtesy of the Cork Examiner.

weatherproof trousers and donning my lifejacket.

We rowed out quickly and boarded **Helen Wycherley**. In minutes the engines were started and mooring chain slipped. At this point when you look down towards the mountainous seas breaking at the bar, you realise this is going to be no picnic and you cannot ask the 'driver' to let you off at the next stop. The wind was blowing severe gale force 11 from the south-east, which makes the bar at Courtmacsherry an unforgiving place.

The Coxswain said, as we passed the old boathouse on our way out, *"everybody inside, all doors closed"*. Myself and two more retreated to the small aft radio cabin to make more room for the experienced hands in the compact wheelhouse.

The sensation of the next few minutes are indelibly etched in my mind. The Watson hit the first breaker with a tremendous force and as she buried herself into the wave a deadening sound came over the boat, except for the sound of the twin propellers digging

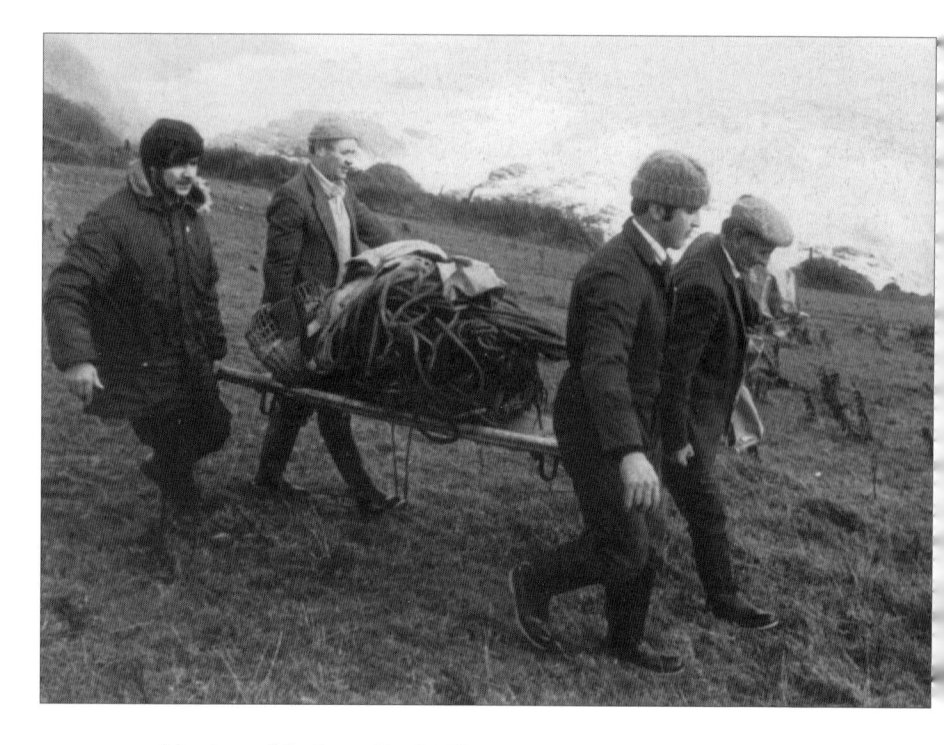

Members of the Seven Heads Lifesaving group arriving at Barry's Point to begin a shore search on the afternoon of Saturday December 19th. 1981.
Photograph courtesy of the Cork Examiner.

into the sea to try and beat the power of the huge waves. The Lifeboat emerged in seconds and flew in mid air to meet the next roller, the noise of the propellers had changed sound dramatically, no slow hum but a wild revving of bronze looking for sea. They didn't have to wait long to get it, the Lifeboat crashed into the trough with a deafening thud sending any loose fittings to the floor of the cabin and shaking everything else mercilessly.

As the Lifeboat buried herself into the next wave my logical brain was trying to work it all out, if this boat weighs up to 22 tons what awesome force can lift us up and send us hurtling through the December air as if we were just a small toy?

Of course, as the years have gone by, I have since come to realise that logic has no place in natures plan as the power of the sea will ever be supreme.

As I looked out through the small porthole in the cabin I struggled to make out the lamp which stands on the headland at the southern side of the harbour mouth. When I caught a momentary glimpse I wondered if I might see it again, lifeboats, though fantastically built, have been no strangers to capsizing. In recent years **Longhope** and **Fraserburgh** in Scotland both capsized on service with large loss of life. These do not make

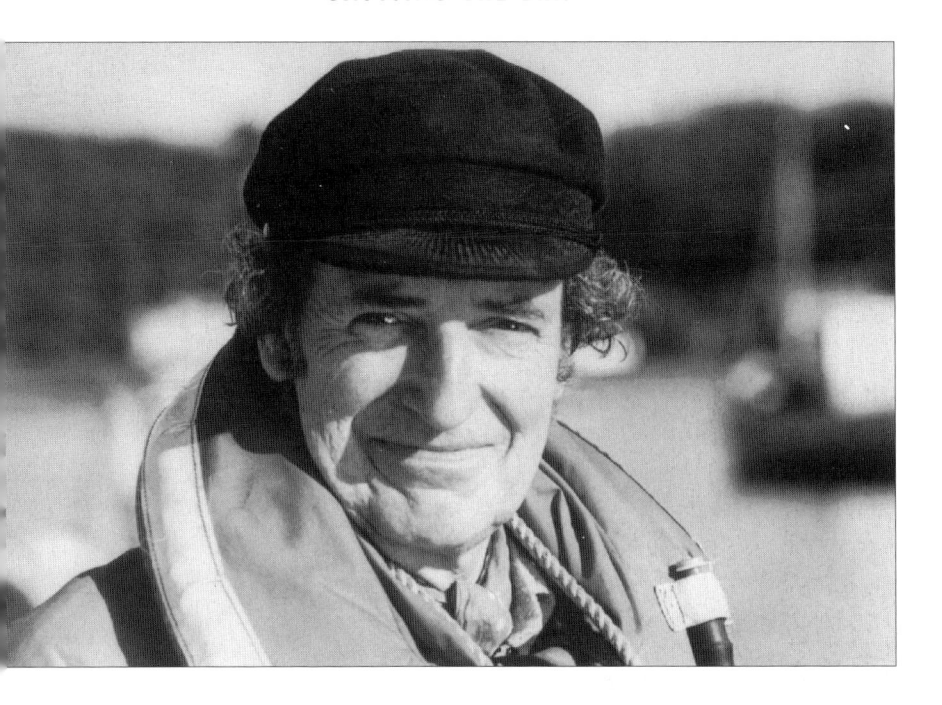

Sammy Mearns who retired in 1980 was coxswain since 1977.
Photograph courtesy of RNLI Poole.

healthy thoughts as you sit in the acrid air of the small cabin and I soon parted with my midday dinner. Beyond the bar the seas were unbelievably rough, though without the slamming. The Coxswain nursed the boat across the bay to Barry's Point. Along the way a sleeping bag and other flotsam were picked up.

Barry's Point itself was a mass of broken water and driving spray. The Lifeboat carried out a big search but nothing was found, with the fading light a helicopter was requested by the Coxswain and a Sea King from R.A.F. Brawdy in Wales arrived. They did a large sweep of the bay in extremely poor visibility but could not find a trace of any survivor from the angling boat. The time was now and as I sat in the cabin with my stomach in turmoil I was amazed at the dexterity of some of my fellow crew in eating soup and chocolate with casual ease. When we concluded the search, the Coxswain decided it would be fool hardy to attempt to re-enter Courtmacsherry harbour with such a large following sea to contend with.

One of the biggest dangers in a Lifeboat is that of a big sea pushing the boat forward so quickly that you lose steering and then lie across the waves, this is called broaching and it is at this point capsize is most likely to occur. Therefore, we had to make the best of it and sit it out at anchor, in Broadstrand, getting as much shelter as possible from under the

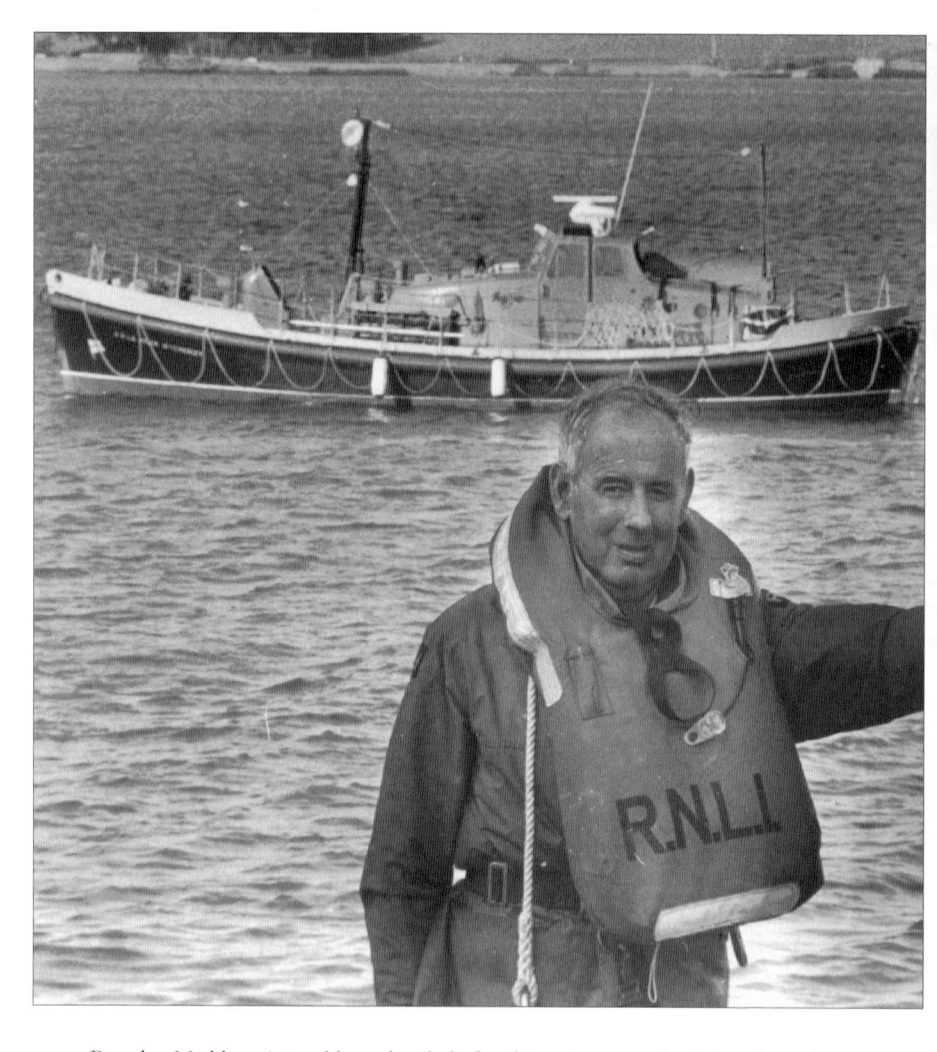

Brendan Madden pictured here shortly before his retirement after 42 year's service on Courtmacsherry Lifeboat. In the background is the **Helen Wycherley**.
Photograph courtesy of John Sheehan Photography.

southern shore. Throughout the afternoon, as well as VHF radio contact with shore, we were in contact on MF radio with the men of Ballycotton lighthouse in east Cork. The keeper, that night, showed what a great service they provided in pre-automation days, by offering to stay up throughout the night and calling up every hour to ensure we were safe.

Regrettably the MF radio brought bad news also. We were not the only Lifeboat at

At a function to mark his retirement Brendan Madden was presented with
a framed certificate of service.
(L to R) Liam Hannigan RNLI hull surveyor, Robbie Robertson RNLI district engineer,
Brendan Madden and Des Bateman Hon. Sec. Courtmacsherry Lifeboat
Photograph courtesy of Michael Minihane.

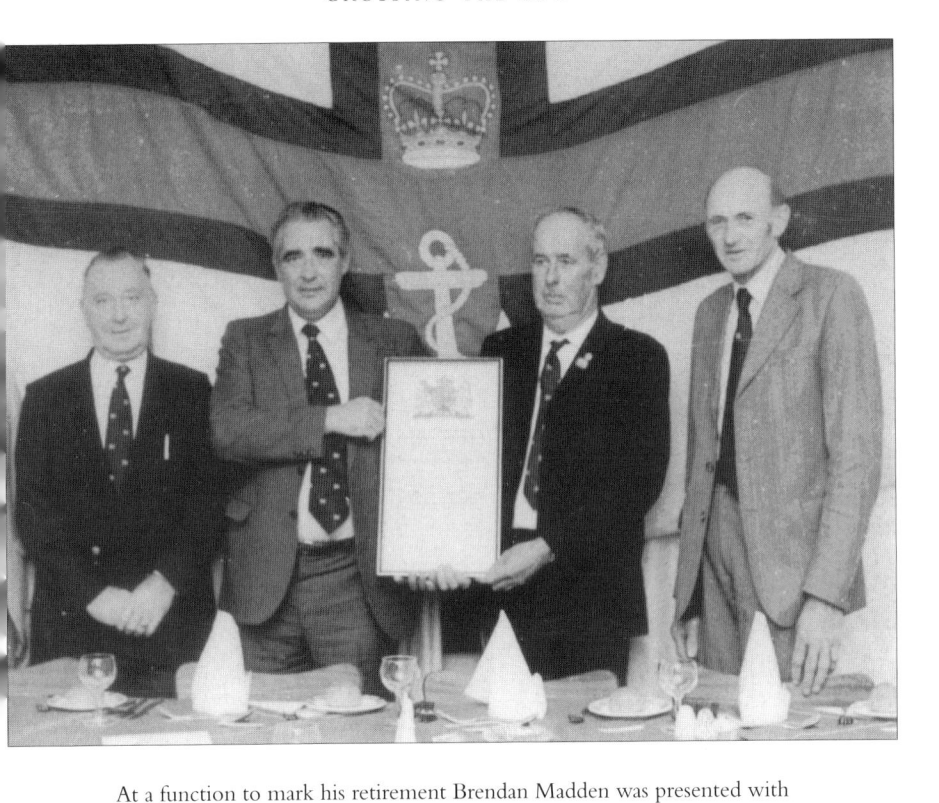

sea. Penlee Lifeboat, in Cornwall,(A Watson, The **Solomon Brown**) was at sea for a much shorter but more tragic launch than ours. She had launched around 8.00 to go to the assistance of a cargo vessel, the **Union Star**, with eight people on board, drifting helplessly ashore on the southern side of the Cornish coast not far from Lands End. At 9.20, having bravely taken off four people from the stricken ship, no more was heard from Penlee Lifeboat or the Union Star. All sixteen people had perished. By 10.00 the radio on our Lifeboat was buzzing with chilling messages that wreckage from the **Solomon Brown** was being washed ashore near Tater Du Lighthouse. It is strange that a place and men whom you never even knew would evoke such sadness amongst us but I suppose its the bond that unites Lifeboatmen everywhere and reminds one that but for the grace of God it could be you. Meanwhile, around the shores of Courtmacsherry Bay, local members of the Coast and Cliff Rescue Service were combing the shoreline for any trace of the missing man.

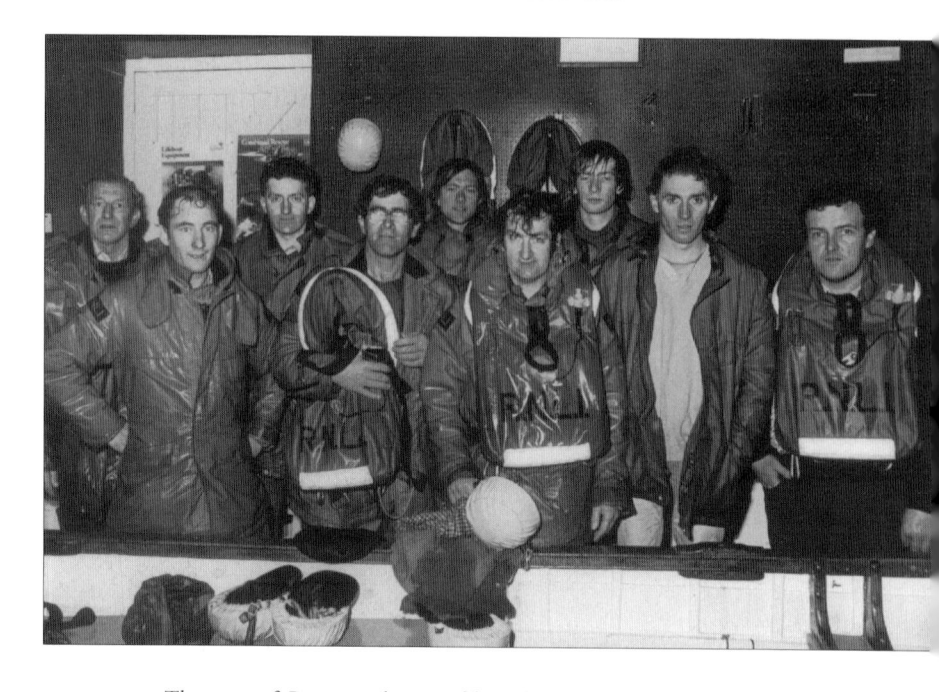

The crew of Courtmacsherry Lifeboat following the service to the ship
Elizabeth of Liberia on November 21st.1984.
(L to R) Thomas Mulcahy, Dan O'Dwyer, Vincent O'Donovan, Cornelius Whelton, Adrian Gannon, Dermot O'Mahony, Colin Bateman, James Brickley and Barry O' Flynn.
Photograph courtesy of the Cork Examiner.

Out at sea, the Lifeboat lay at anchor with engines running, until dawn, when the anchor was hauled up and the dangerous trip for home begun. The fury of the night's gale had abated somewhat but the entrance to the harbour was still a foul looking prospect due to the massive swell. Accordingly the drogue was trailed out to prevent the Lifeboat from broaching and the **Helen Wycherley** slipped back into the gentle waters of Courtmacsherry harbour tying up to the pier to refuel at 9.00am. All that day shore parties were out in force to check all parts of the bay but for their efforts all that was recovered was bits of wreckage. A month later the fishing boat was salvaged and brought to Courtmacsherry pier where the fisherman's body was recovered within. For this service a framed Letter of Thanks signed by the Duke of
, Chairman of The Institution, was presented to second Coxswain, Brendan Madden.

During the '80's we saw a further decline in the population of the locality with a short tourism season becoming of major importance to the local economy. The R.N.L.I. locally also witnessed the retirement of two of its former Coxswains.

Brendan Madden retired in May 1983, after giving forty two years service. It would probably take a book on its own to adequately cover such a long and dedicated service. Brendan joined the Lifeboat as a crewman when he was only seventeen years of age and was appointed full time motor mechanic in 1966, a position he held up to the time of his retirement. He was also acting Coxswain during 1982. He had seen major changes in his time in the type of Lifeboat used, to the advent of radar and more efficient radio communcations. Upon Brendan's retirement, Thomas Mulcahy was appointed motor mechanic.

Sammy Mearns' retirement in January 1982 brought to an end his ten year involvement, having been a crewman from 1972 - 74, then second Coxswain, 1974 -76 before becoming Coxswain in 1977. Sammy was Coxswain on the fateful night in 1979 during the Fastnet race. It is a touch ironic that Sammy Mearns, who bought and renovated the Old Coastguard Station, overlooking the village, should have become part of the history of Courtmacsherry R.N.L.I. since it was the original coastguards who played such an active role 150 years previously.

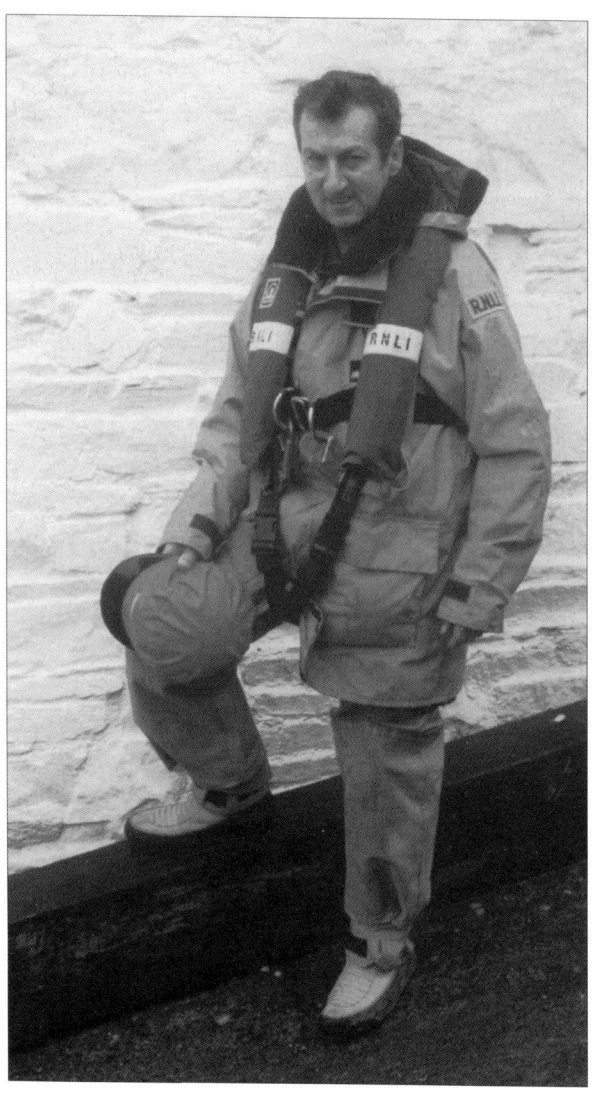

Dermot O' Mahony coxswain of Courtmacsherry Lifeboat since 1984, has been on the crew since 1962.
Photograph courtesy of Martin Walsh.

Taking over as Coxswain in late 1982 was Dermot O'Mahony who, though he will

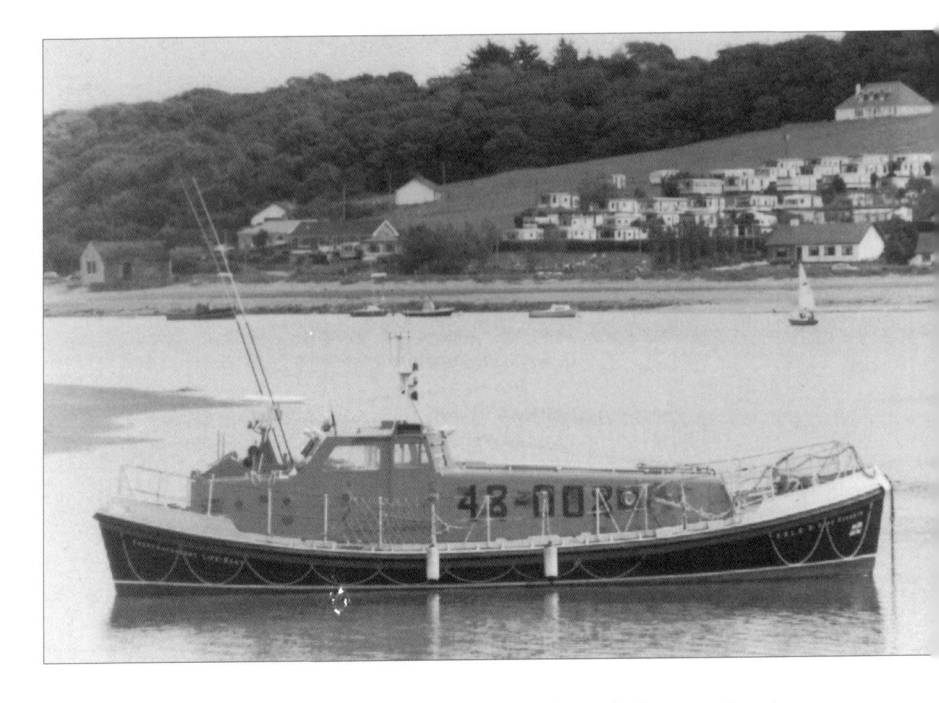

The Solent class Lifeboat **R. Hope Roberts** which was stationed
in Courtmacsherry from 1987 – 1993.

Photograph courtesy of Martin Walsh.

not thank me for calling him a veteran, has been involved with Courtmacsherry Lifeboat since 1962. Dermot, who is the Master of a Tug working on the Shannon estuary, had previously been in Bantry Bay and sailed the world as a cadet with Irish Shipping. In spite of working away from home he had the clever knack of being around for some of the major services including the Fastnet Race and the unsuccessful search in December 1981.

One of the roughest services upon taking up the Coxswain's role was on the 21st November 1984 when the **Elizabeth** a 118,000 ton cargo vessel reported that he had a sick crewman on board who needed evacuation. The Lifeboat left harbour at 14.40 to rendezvous with the vessel off the Seven Heads. The wind was severe storm force 9 and a huge sea running. Shortly after 4.00pm, the **Helen Wycherley** was manoeuvred on the lee side to run with the **Elizabeth** as she steamed easterly. The crewman was lowered by rope from what seemed like a six storey building gently on to the deck of the Lifeboat. **Helen Wycherley** then headed back for Courtmacsherry harbour where an ambulance was waiting.

Perhaps even in this testing work humour can sometimes surface, so it was when the ambulance crew boarded the Lifeboat at the pier. On enquiring as to the condition of the patient, *"which patient ?"* came the reply from a doctor who had been Volunteered to travel with the Lifeboat and had been forced to adopt a horizontal position not long after leaving harbour.

In June 1985, Air India flight 182 crashed into the sea about 100 miles south west of Mizen Head. Courtmacsherry Lifeboat was launched and headed west as far as Baltimore to refuel but, by then, it was apparent that there were no survivors so the **Sir Godfrey Baring**, on relief duty, returned to Courtmacsherry.

October 1987 saw **Helen Wycherley** sail off into retirement after her eighteen years glorious service in Courtmacsherry. She was purchased by a businessman in Crosshaven where she was put into service as an angling boat. The replacement lifeboat marked another dramatic change. The **R.Hope Roberts** was a Solent class steel hulled boat with aluminium wheelhouse and superstructure, this made the boat inherently self righting. Originally built by Camper Nicholson, in the Isle of Wight, for Rosslare in 1969, she subsequently moved to Fraserburgh in Scotland from 1979 to 1985. On again to Galway Bay until the spring of 1987. The Lifeboat was overhauled at Skinners Boatyard in Baltimore and her arrival was warmly welcomed at Courtmacsherry where the crew were eager to continue her tremendous lifesaving record.

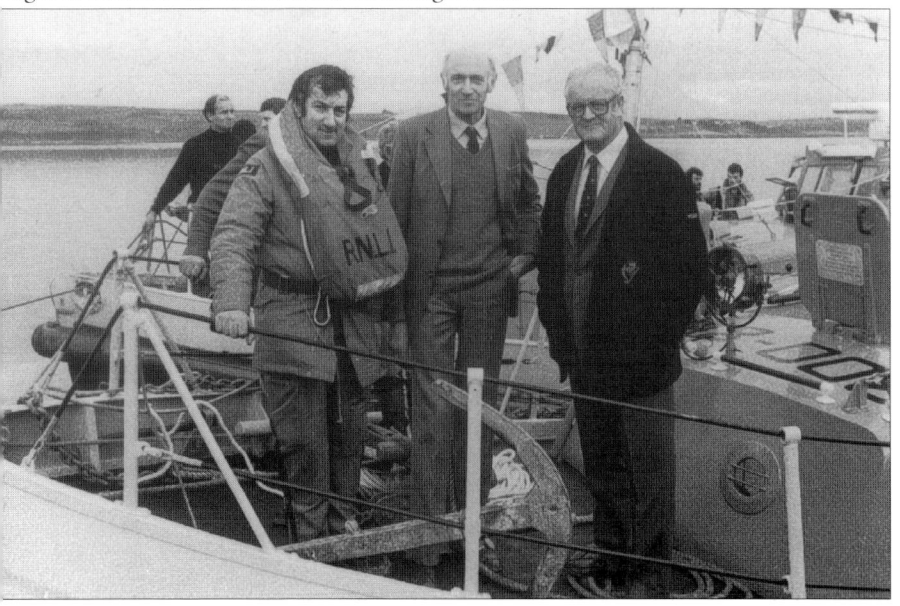

Pictured on Saturday November 28th,1987 when the **R.Hope Roberts** was Blessed and re-dedicated in a ceremony at Courtmacsherry pier.
(L to R)Dermot O'Mahony (cox.) Des Bateman (Hon Sec) Clayton Love Jnr. a member of the RNLI committee of management.
Photograph courtesy of the Cork Examiner.

CHAPTER 15
TOWARDS 2000
1990 – 1995

Then they cry unto the Lord in their trouble, and he bringeth them
out of their distresses.
He maketh the storm a calm, so that the waves thereof are still.
Then are they glad because they be quiet; so he bringeth them unto
their desired haven.

From Psalm 107, Verses 23--30

As we move swiftly into the high tech era, the demands on the Lifeboat service remain the same. At 7.30am on July 23rd, 1991 when the bleeper shook me from my sound sleep with a message that a yacht was on fire off the Seven Heads, I didn't really take much notice of the message as I hurriedly dressed to dash out and head for the boathouse. **R. Hope Roberts** slipped her moorings at 7.45am and motored out of the harbour. The sea was choppy with the wind blowing about force five. Radio contact with the casualty, **Karma**, was soon established and using VHF direction finding, we were soon alongside the forty foot yacht. The crew told us of their plight, they had an engine electrical fire and then their rudder broke. At that point they decided to call the Lifeboat. The yacht was safely tied up at the pier by 11.15a.m. and the Lifeboat re-fuelled and put back on her moorings by 11.45 a.m. All fairly simple and straight-forward no medal today anyway!

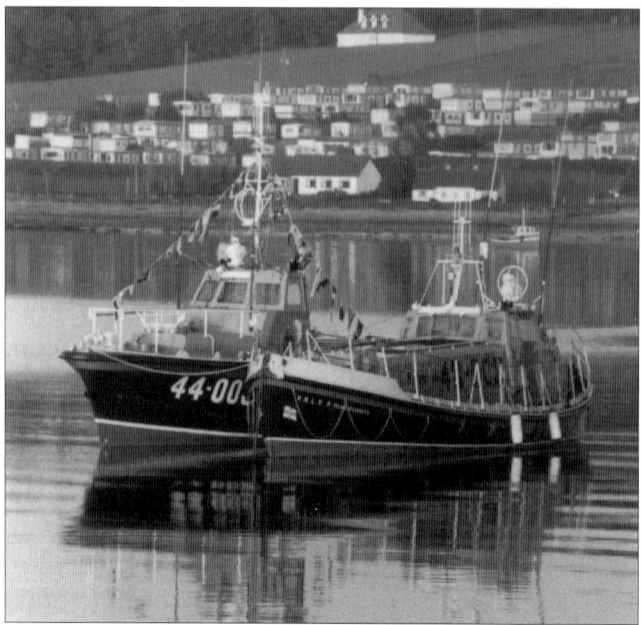

However, as the day progressed the Customs took a keen interest in the vessel and

May 1993 and the **Arthur and Blanche Harris** is moored outside the soon to depart **R. Hope Roberts**

Photograph courtesy of Martin Walsh.

80

discovered half a ton of cannabis resin in 25 individual bales on board the yacht. The drugs would have a street value of £7.5 million. The pier was, by now, a bustling thoroughfare with Gardaí, Customs, Reporters and T.V. crews mingling with a mass of sightseers. Yes, Sam Goldwyn was right, everyone is famous for ten seconds!

The station was anticipating news of a replacement for **R.Hope Roberts** since the R.N.L.I. had pledged to have an all fast fleet by 1993. Several of the crew had gone to Dunmore East in 1992 to view the prototype Trent class which was visiting the Irish coast as part of her trials and evaluation. We all came home that day very impressed and could not wait to get our hands on one of our own. That was to come soon but, in the meantime, a Waveney was allocated to the station pending the arrival of the Trent.

As a crew, we got double value out of that as we had to take the boat from Arklow, where it had been overhauled, to Poole and following crew training, back home to Courtmacsherry. The passage there and back gives the crew a great introduction to the boat and calls at places like Milford Haven, Falmouth, Brixham, Newlyn and Salcombe does you no harm either! The ***Arthur and Blanche Harris*** was originally built for Barry Dock, Wales in 1968 and was a 44 foot steel hulled boat with aluminium superstructure. Capable of up to 13 knots and self righting, in the event of capsize, she would be a good

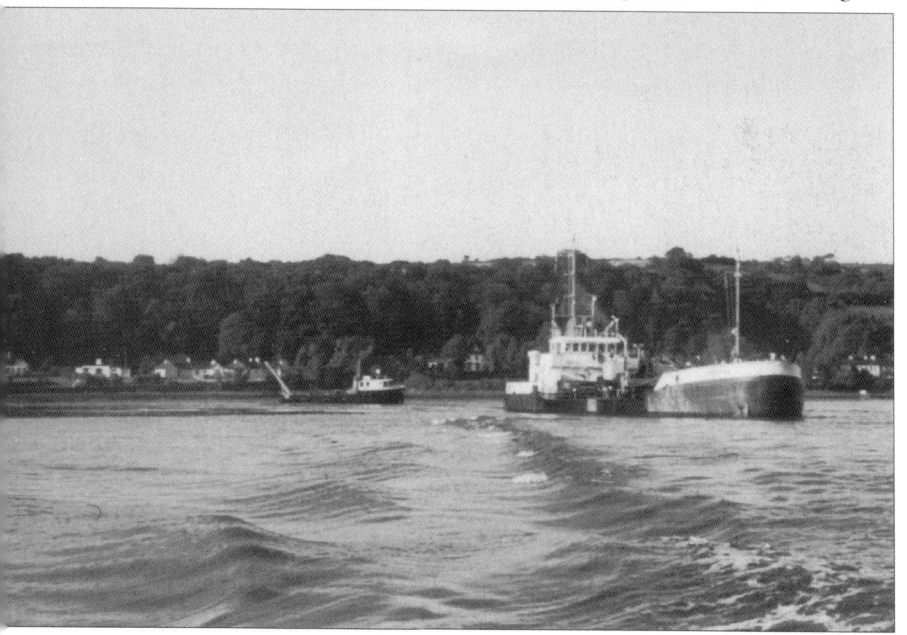

The dredging of the channel in Courtmacsherry harbour underway in 1993.
Photograph courtesy of Michael Cox.

stepping stone to the Trent. ***Arthur and Blanche Harris*** had come to Courtmacsherry with a rich pedigree having launched two hundred and seventy seven times and saved one hundred and eleven lives so far. ***R. Hope Roberts*** sailed off to Poole in June 1993 to be sold, eventually being shipped to Australia to continue her lifesaving work with a voluntary group there.

In 1993 too the long awaited dredging of the channel in Courtmacsherry harbour was completed which would ensure that the Lifeboat and fishing boats could get in and out of the harbour at all stages of the tide. The R.N.L.I. itself committed £50,000 to the fund, the rest of which was subscribed locally, by the Department of the Marine and by local authority contributions.

1995 will be a momentous occasion in the stations long and varied history when the ***Frederick Storey Cockburn*** Lifeboat goes into service. Built at Osborne's, Littlehampton, she is a superb craft, slightly over fourteen metres in length (46 feet 9 inches), made from fibre reinforced composite material. Powered by two 808h.p. M.A.N. diesel engines, carrying nearly 950 gallons of fuel she can reach speeds of up to 25 knots which gives a

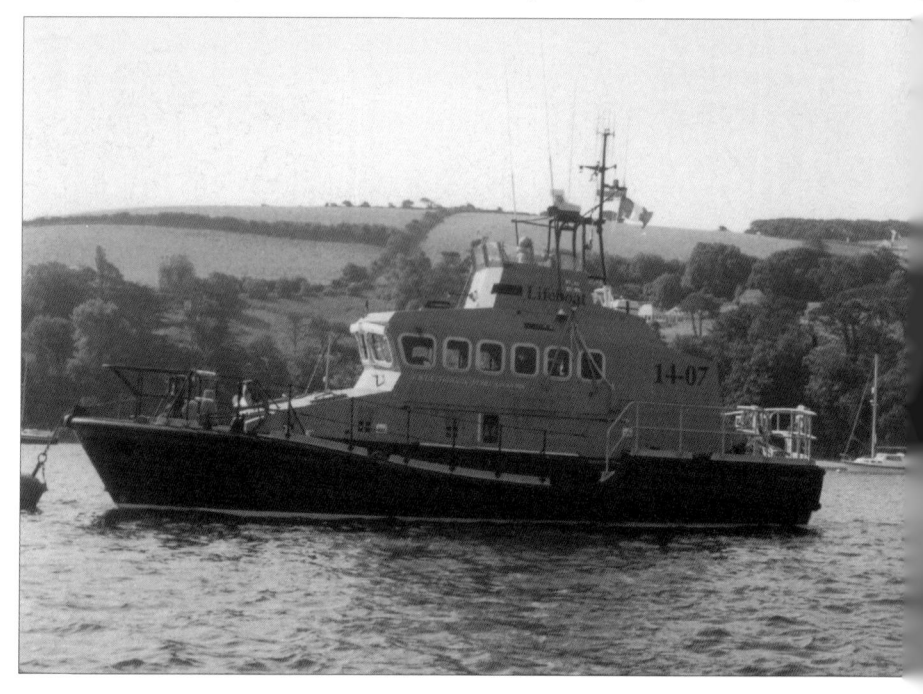

Courtmacsherry's magnificent new Lifeboat, ***Fredrick Storey Cockburn*** (O.N. 1205) at anchor in Salcombe Harbour, South Devon during the 40 hour trials of the boat's machinery in June 1995.

Photograph courtesy of Michael Cox.

...ange of 250 miles at top speed. Equipped with a dazzling array of equipment including all the latest navigational aids such as daylight radar, chart plotter and satellite navigation it should prove a tremendous improvement to the search and rescue capabilities of the Courtmacsherry Lifeboat. Amongst the fine equipment fitted to the new Lifeboat is a microwave oven to further add to the crew's culinary expertise!. This craft, costing over £1,000,000 has seating for the six crew and also for a doctor when required on service. As part of her trials, the lifeboat was turned upside down by crane in December 1994 on the water adjacent to the boatyard. The straps from the crane were then slipped and the Lifeboat came back upright in a matter of seconds. The greater part of the massive cost of this magnificent boat has been funded from a legacy of the late Mr. Fredrick Storey Cockburn of Worthing in Sussex .

The Waveney class that he replaces will serve in the relief fleet for a while before being sold off.

Several of the crew have been on trials with the new boat in June 1995 and to Poole, Headquarters, in August to undergo extensive training both in the classroom and afloat. It is with tremendous pride that the crew sailed up the harbour on August 24th after a successful training passage from England. The crew and local committee are looking forward now to the reconstruction of the lifeboat house. The new facility will mean improved drying facilities for the protective clothing, toilets and a shower

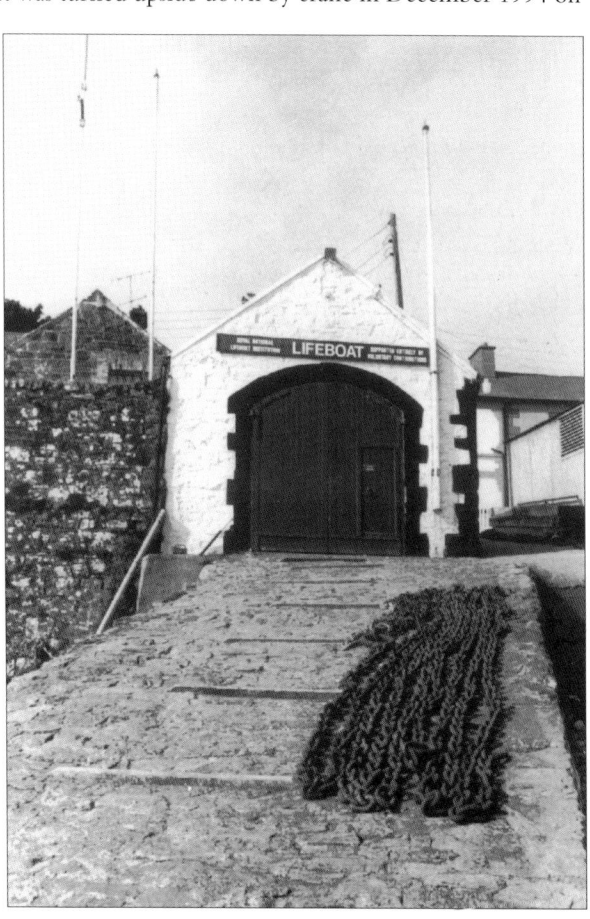

The Lifeboat House as it is today viewed from the slipway down which many a Courtmacsherry man has ran in haste to board the Lifeboats that have been stationed here.

Photograph courtesy of Martin Walsh

and a new crew room which may be used for meetings or lectures.

The R.N.L.I. have allocated funds for the improvement of shore facilities at many stations around the coast and we, at Courtmacsherry, look forward eagerly to the welcome improvement. The decade, so far, has seen Courtmacsherry Lifeboat launch over sixty times.

The Lifeboat crew as ever, even as you read this, are ready and waiting to go to sea to help anyone in peril. Just the same as they have since 1825 – long may it continue.

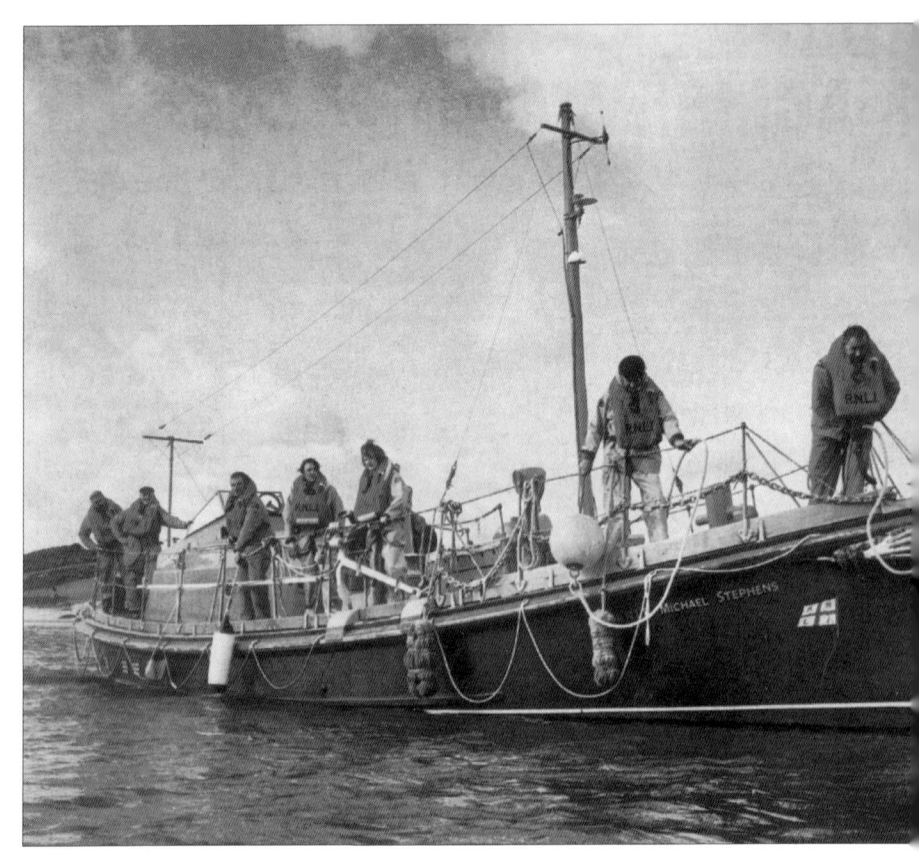

This photograph of the relief Lifeboat **Michael Stephens** was published in colour in the Cork Holly Bough in December 1974.
Pictured (L to R) Tony Dorman, Paddy Keohane, Thomas Mulcahy, John Hodnett, Noel Fleming, Sammy Mearns and Brendan Madden.

CHAPTER 16
FOR THOSE IN PERIL..........
A BRIEF HISTORY OF THE R.N.L.I.

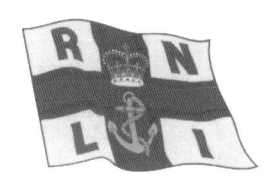

THE R.N.L.I. itself is but a year older than Courtmacsherry Lifeboat having been founded in 1824. The seeds for it's formation were sown some years earlier. The Netherlands government, in January 12, 1769, issued a decree for the setting up of a Lifeboat service at six places along the Dutch coast. This probably was Europe's first Lifeboat service. In Britain too about this time, concern was growing at various locations about the lack of suitable boats for rescue work, this concern being further heightened by a major sea tragedy in 1789. In March of that year a ship named *Adventure* ran ashore at the mouth of the river Tyne in a violent storm. Onlookers had gathered in their thousands and offered local boatmen rewards to save the crew but, none would venture out as, to do so on such a day, would have meant certain death.

The sight of men being swept away one by one awakened the nation and provided the spur to have Lifeboats provided at various points around the coast. Members of a social club in South Shields, known as the Gentlemen of the Lawe House, offered a two guinea prize for the best Lifeboat design. Many entries were received and much debate has gone on as to who the winner was, but suffice to say, that a combination of designs submitted by William Wouldhave, a parish clerk, and Henry Greathead, a boat builder, both of the locality, was subsequently built by Greathead. This Lifeboat was appropriately called the *Original* since she was the first boat built as a Lifeboat and not a conversion. It was 30 feet long with twelve oars and had seven cwt. of cork for buoyancy. After launching in 1789, she served for forty years at the mouth of the river Tyne. They could scarcely have known what a great service to seafarers they had begun.

Several more of these Lifeboats were built by Greathead for various places on the U.K. coast and each operated independently. Similarly, a lifeboat operated at Douglas Bay, on the Isle of Man, since 1802. A famous man, Sir William Hillary, lived there and was a crew member on many rescues resulting in his being awarded, no less than, three gold medals. Sir William, recognising the lack of organisation and the consequent gaps in lifeboat cover, wrote an historic *Appeal to the Nation* in 1823. In his appeal he pointed out the loss to the nation from shipwreck and the untold heartache caused by the unnecessary deaths and the effect this too was having on the morale of all seamen. The effects of Sir

William Hillary's appeal was immediate, wide sympathy and support was gained.

One of those impressed by Hillary's appeal was Thomas Wilson M.P. who also had a business in London. He called a meeting at the City of London Tavern on 12th February 1824, at which it was agreed that a national organisation should be formed to preserve life from shipwreck. A further meeting was held three weeks later on 4th March. 1824 at which the National Institution for the Preservation of the Life from Shipwreck was formed. The original Chairman was Thomas Wilson M.P. with King George 4th as patron and the then Prime Minister as President.

The Institution changed it's name to the Royal National Lifeboat Institution in 1854 The Lifeboat service in Ireland has been provided by the R.N.L.I. since 1824 also Apparently the R.N.L.I. asked the new Free State Government if they had any problem with their continuing providing the service and they, quite rightly, said they didn't and so it has remained ever since.

The R.N.L.I. today is a complex organisation with over two hundred lifeboat stations all over the coast of the U.K. and Ireland with stations in diverse places from Alderney in the Channel Islands to Lerwick, in the Shetlands, or Kilronan, in the Aran Islands. With new Lifeboats, similar to the magnificent Trent Class, constantly being built, at a cost well in excess of one million pounds, voluntary financial contributions are still the R.N.L.I.'s only source of income. This voluntary system has proven itself over one hundred and seventy years to be the most efficient way of providing a Lifeboat service. Contributions vary from bequests of millions to 50pence pieces, given at a flag day, all are equally well received.

Due to population imbalance, the cost of running the Lifeboats of the Irish coast cannot be met solely from funds collected in Ireland. Therefore, the balance is contributed by central funds in England. Locally, the station is administered by The Honorary Secretary and Committee. Now, the Honorary Secretary, at each station, does more than just write letters. It is he who manages the local station and must authorise every launch of the lifeboat. This will mean, perhaps, getting out of bed in the middle of the night and activating the pagers and driving to the station to convey all the particulars to the Coxswain and crew as they don their gear. Often the Honorary Secretary will stay in radio contact with the boat to ensure that any further updated information may be passed directly to the crew of the Lifeboat. It is after the call, some will say, that the real work starts for the Honorary Secretary, the paperwork, with all the details of times and tides, weather and sea, and crew members names are all filled in for despatching to H.Q.

The crews too everywhere, as in Courtmacsherry, are volunteers, giving of their time freely, not only to go to the aid of the seafarer in distress, but, for the many exercises and training courses, which are required to be efficient in operating a complex craft such a **Frederick Storey Cockburn** now stationed here. Each station has a full time mechanic whose job it is to ensure that the boat is kept in constant readiness for service. The volunteer crew do get a nominal payment to, in some small way, compensate them for any loss of earnings they may incur while on a Lifeboat call.

The R.N.L.I. headquarters is in Poole, Dorset, on the south coast of England. It is from there that spares of all types are despatched from a complete engine to a first aid kit. It is there also that the training centre is located. This building, right on the waterfront, is where all crew training is carried out before sailing back home with any new boat. "*Who calls the Lifeboat*"? is a constant question and it has a variety of answers. In Ireland, the situation is as follows. In most cases nowadays, a vessel will usually have a VHF radio through which he may pass his distress message to a coast radio station which is also a marine rescue sub-centre. The operator there will check the chart and verify which Lifeboat would best be able to offer assistance. He will then telephone the Honorary Secretary to inform him of the nature of the distress and all relevant particulars.

The Honorary Secretary can immediately activate the crew's electronic pagers and shortly the Lifeboat will be under way. A system is presently being installed that will allow the crew to be paged directly by Marine Rescue Co-ordination Centres (M.R.C.C.), though the Honorary Secretary must still approve the launch.

A vessel in trouble can also use a red flare to attract attention which is hopefully spotted by someone ashore who will dial 999 or the Honorary Secretary direct. The launch is then put in motion. Of course, another vessel may receive a distress message or see a flare or some other sign of trouble, in this situation that ship can pass on the information by radio. Several lifeboats calls, every year, are initiated by a local person who may be anxious about a family member or friend who has gone fishing or boating hours previously and at nightfall still has not returned. Many of these people will telephone one of the crew and they, in turn, can contact the Honorary Secretary to authorise a launch.

Search and Rescue work in Ireland these days may also involve other agencies who work in close harmony with Lifeboats. These are:- In the air, the helicopters of the Air Corps, Department of the Marine helicopter based at Shannon and the R.A.F. On the ground, the Department of the Marine organised Coast and Cliff Rescue Service, the Gardai, Civil Defence and the Irish Red Cross and on the sea the Naval Service. Together, they provide one of the best services to mariners of all types anywhere in the world.

The history of the R.N.L.I. itself is but a mirror of that of Courtmacsherry Lifeboat. The constant evolution of technology has meant that boats have gone from a humble rowing boat up to today's craft with 1700 engine horse power available and all the most modern navigational equipment on board. There is, though, a common thread that links all the decades, the sea is an ever present danger to those who use it, for pleasure or profit, no amount of technology can ever control it. The crews that man each and every Lifeboat are aware of that, even if it is in the dark recesses of the mind, yet they are prepared to go and face it whatever may prevail.

May the spirit that has carried the R.N.L.I. for over 170 years long continue to do so.

APPENDICES

APPENDIX 1

ALL SERVICES BY THE LIFEBOATS STATIONED AT COURTMACSHERRY

Unfortunately no records exist for the period 1825 to 1869, however two rescues are recorded during that period when shore boats were used

21.02.1840	Sloop **John and Ellen** shipwrecked at entrance to harbour	The crew of 4 were rescued

The R.N.L.I. Silver medal was awarded to Lt. B. E. Quadling of the Coastguards for leading this rescue

07.02.1842	A brig **Latona** wrecked off Courtmacsherry	14 crew rescued.

The R. N. L. I. Gold medal was awarded to Lt. B. E. Quadling for his part in this rescue. This is the only gold medal so far awarded to Courtmacsherry.

City of Dublin Lifeboat.

30.08.1869	Brigantine **Wave of York** ran ashore having developed a leak	Crew rescued by fishing boat.
01.02.1870	**Osborne** Reported in trouble at the barrels.	Vessel anchored and in no danger
14.10.1871	Schooner **Helen Lass** of Aberystwyth drifted ashore at Garrettstown	Vessel gone safely up on shore crew all safe.
09.01.1875	Steamer **Abbotsford** of Liverpool broken down near Dunworley.	Vessel taken in tow by another ship.
12.02.1875	Barque **Hattie B** of Liverpool disabled and anchored at Black Tom rock.	Lifeboat stood by until tow arrived.
28.12.1876	Schooner in trouble at Barry'scove.	Vessel had sailed out of danger before Lifeboat got there.
22.10.1877	Ship in distress off Garrettstown.	Nothing found, probably sailed out of danger.

12.01.1879	Barque **General Caulfield** of Newcastle, wrecked at mouth of Courtmacsherry harbour	18 men rescued by Lifeboat.
22.01.1879	A large ship **Nelson** in difficulties off the 7 heads.	Ship had sailed safely west before the Lifeboat got there
10.02.1881	Unknown barque thought to be in trouble on the Barrel rocks.	The ship had sailed away east before the Lifeboat reached her
03.03.1881	A brig **Coleridge** of Newcastle ran ashore near Dunworley	Lifeboat was on the way by road but recalled.
30.11.1881	A steamer **Glen Devon** of Leith in trouble off 7 heads.	Lifeboat stood by for a while, tug towed ship to safety.
02.01.1883	Unknown barque thought to be in difficulties off the 7 heads.	Ship sailed away as the Lifeboat approached
04.06.1883	Cutter yacht **Kingston** of Cork drifting ashore at Broadstrand.	Owner refused help and sailed safely away.
23.01.1884	Schooner **Hebe** of Cork in distress at Broadstrand.	Lifeboat ran out anchors for her.

The Farrant Lifeboat (O.N. 103)

T*he system of official numbers (O.N.) was introduced in 1887 and the Farrant was the first Courtmacsherry Lifeboat to get a number.*

17.05.1886	Fishing smack **Harry** of Courtmacsherry in trouble off Broadstrand.	Lifeboat escorted her safely into harbour.
15.08.1886	A ship **Windaw** of Liverpool on Cow rock in Dunworley bay.	The crew got safely ashore themselves.
12.11.1891	Ship **Gylfe** went ashore on the Old Head of Kinsale.	Ship completely wrecked before Lifeboat arrived.
03.08.1898	**Ecclefechan** of Glasgow ashore at Dunworley.	Lifeboat stood by.
20.07.1900	A steamer **Texan** of Liverpool holed in a collision off the 7 heads.	Lifeboat stood by until tugs arrived
14.01.1901	Report of a steamer in trouble in the bay.	Lifeboat not required.

The Kezia Gwilt Lifeboat (O. N. 467)

07.03.1902	Report of vessel in difficulties near inner Barrels.	False alarm.
01.01.1904	French barque **Faulconnier** wrecked at Travarra.	11 of the crew taken off by the Lifeboat.
08.11.1908	Steamer **Queen** disabled East of the Old Head of Kinsale.	Lifeboat went as far as the Old Head but her assistance not required.
19.11.1909	Report of a ship in trouble in the bay.	Lifeboat launched but no trace found.
18.02.1910	Italian barque **F.S. Ciampa** wrecked at Dunworley all 25 crew perished.	Lifeboat launched but couldn't get there due to gale.
07.02.1911	Ketch reported in difficulties West of the Galley Head.	Lifeboat went as far as the Galley but a steamer had towed ketch safely East.
22.04.1911	Barque **Falls of Garry** of Glasgow ashore near Oysterhaven.	Lifeboat went to scene but her help not required.
22.07.1912	Report of steamer ashore at Dunworley.	False alarm so Lifeboat returned.
09.07.1914	Steamer **S. S. Nith** of Maryport ashore in Dunworley Bay.	Crew had got safely ashore when Lifeboat arrived.
07.05.1915	Passenger liner **Lusitania** torpedoed off the Old Head of Kinsale.	Lifeboat helped in the recovery of bodies.
21.05.1918	American destroyer on rocks at 7 heads.	She had got off before the Lifeboat arrived.
02.12.1918	Tanker **Konakry** went ashore at Garrettstown following a collision.	All crew had got ashore before Lifeboat arrived.
14.03.1919	Sloop of war reported in trouble off the 7 heads.	False alarm, Lifeboat returned.

The Sarah Ward and William David Crossweller Lifeboat
(O. N. 716)

27.10.1930	Report of a vessel on fire 4 miles S E of the Galley Head.	A search carried out , nothing found.
27.06.1931	Ketch **Ivy P** drifting onto rocks at the Galley Head.	Lifeboat towed her off and she proceeded safely.
08.12.1932	Schooner **Elizabeth Drew** in trouble off Garrettstown	Lifeboat escorted her to Courtmacsherry.
11.12.1932	Liner **Viking Star** broken down off Galley Head.	Lifeboat went to scene, assistance not required.
19.01.1933	Small coaster **Hibernia** on rocks at entrance to harbour.	Lifeboat took off 3 crew.
20.08.1934	Yacht **Mab** ashore at entrance to harbour.	Lifeboat went to scene, but 3 crew had swam ashore.
21.06.1936	Steam trawler **Point Castle** of Swansea aground on Old Head of Kinsale.	Lifeboat stood by until refloated.
24.06.1938	Spanish trawler **Baron of Vigo** aground and sunk on the Old Head of Kinsale.	Lifeboat stood by while crew transferred to sister ship.
18.03.1939	Fishing vessel broken down off the Old Head of Kinsale.	Lifeboat searched but she had reached Courtmacsherry after engine repairs.
15.03.1939	Oil Tanker **British Influence** of London torpedoed 250 miles off Fastnet.	42 crew brought to Courtmacsherry by Lifeboat from passing ship.
16.06.1939	Oil Tanker **Cheyenne** of Newcastle torpedoed off Fastnet.	Lifeboat went West and landed 37 crew in Baltimore.
24.09.1939	Cargo ship **Hayleside** of Newcastle on Tyne shelled and sunk off Cape Clear	Lifeboat searched but another boat took survivors to Schull.

04.01.1940	Cargo vessel **Athelbeach** of Liverpool on rocks at Galley Head.	Lifeboat searched stood by and ran out anchors for ship pending arrival of tugs.
10.07.1940	Drifting empty ship's Lifeboat	Towed to Courtmacsherry.
19.11.1940	Two drifting ships Lifeboats.	Lifeboat searched but found nothing.
20.11.1940	Drifting ships Lifeboat.	Searched but not located.
02.12.1940	Trawler **Kilgerran Castle** of Swansea shelled 25 miles s.w. of Old Head of Kinsale.	Lifeboat went to the scene but crew taken on board other trawlers.

The City of Bradford Lifeboat (O.N. 680)
(On Relief Duty)

| 05.04.1941 | Trawler **Ixeus** broken down in Clonakilty Bay. | Assistance not required. |

The Sarah Ward and William David Crossweller Lifeboat
(O.N. 716)

31.05.1941	Steamer in difficulties at Newfoundland Bay near Cork Harbour.	Ship had got away before Lifeboat arrived.
02.11.1941	Trawler bombed 17 miles south of Seven Heads.	Lifeboat arrived but survivors had been picked up by another trawler.
16.11.1941	Trawler **Dandola** of Aberdeen with engine trouble S-E. of the Old Head of Kinsale.	Lifeboat stood by while another trawler towed her to Kinsale.
24.04.1942	Report of rubber dinghy adrift off Seven Heads.	Search carried out but nothing found.

The City of Bradford Lifeboat (O.N. 680)
(On Relief Duty)

| 13.07.1942 | Motor boat **Shirken** broken down off Oysterhaven. | Boat located and towed to Oysterhaven. |

The Sarah Ward and William David Crossweller Lifeboat
(O.N. 716)

11.08.1944	Missing rowing boat out of Oysterhaven.	Lifeboat recalled while on her way to search.
01.09.1944	Lobster boat **Margaret** of Skibbereen broken down near Howe Strand.	Lifeboat towed her to Courtmacsherry.
13.09.1944	Report of Aeroplane missing between Old Head of Kinsale and Cork Harbour.	Search carried out nothing found.
13.03.1945	Submarine U-260 sunk 5 miles west of Galley Head.	37 of a crew landed at Courtmacsherry.
27.07.1945	Trawler **Flow** reported sunk off Cork Harbour.	Search carried out , nothing found.
29.03.1946	Steamer reported ashore at Galley Head.	Lifeboat carried out a search but nothing found.
18.07.1946	Sailing dinghy overdue out of Courtmacsherry	Boat turned up as Lifeboat was about to search
22.07.1946	Rowing boat with 2 on board overdue	All safe, Lifeboat recalled
28.08.1946	6 sailing boats swept out to sea, report of 1 boy missing.	Search carried out but boy was safely ashore.
21.11.1946	Sand barges in difficulty at the mouth of the harbour.	Lifeboat towed them to safety.
06.11.1947	Report of trawler in distress off Old Head of Kinsale.	Search carried out.
14.04.1948	A motor launch broken down in Courtmacsherry Bay with 5 on board.	Towed to Harbour by Lifeboat.
03.06.1948	Rowing boat with 1 man on board blown out to sea.	Located 7 miles out, and towed to harbour.

| 15.08.1948 | Sailing yacht **Quireda** in danger of going onto rocks at Harbour entrance. | Towed to safety by Lifeboat. |

The Agnes Cross Lifeboat (O.N. 663)
(On Relief Duty)

| 20.08.1948 | Motor boat with 6 on board overdue. | Search carried out and boat escorted to Courtmacsherry. |
| 22.08.1948 | Empty motor launch drifted onto rocks at Dunworley. | Lifeboat went to scene but was too late to save her. |

The Sarah Ward and William David Crossweller Lifeboat
(O.N. 716)

| 15.09.1948 | Trawler in distress near Baltimore | Search carried out but casualty had reached Baltimore. |

The Agnes Cross Lifeboat (O.N.663)
(On Relief Duty)

| 24.05.1949 | A trawler sunk 50 miles W S/W of the Old Head of Kinsale. | Lifeboat went to the spot but crew were rescued by French trawler. |

The Sarah Ward and William David Crossweller Lifeboat
(O.N. 716)

30.07.1950	Boat capsized at Garrettstown 3 people drowned.	Lifeboat went but recalled.
05.05.1952	Plane reported gone into sea off Old Head of Kinsale.	Search carried out, nothing found.
08.11.1952	Small motor boat overdue at Kinsale.	Boat turned up just as lifeboat were heading to area.
28.03.1953	Rowing tender from cargo boat with 3 aboard lost in fog at harbour mouth	Lifeboat towed it to pier.
21.05.1954	Report of small rowing boat missing in Clonakilty Bay.	Search carried out but nothing found.

18.07.1954	Woman fell over cliff at Garrettstown.	Lifeboat recalled.
15.01.1955	Vessel reported in difficulties 10 miles south east of Seven Heads.	Search carried out but nothing found.

The William and Harriot Lifeboat (O.N. 718)
(On Relief Duty)

04.06.1955	Fishing Vessel missing off the Old Head of Kinsale.	Lifeboat searched but vessel had reached port safely.

The Sarah Ward and William David Crossweller Lifeboat (O.N. 716)

02.11.1955	**S.S. Marioute M** of London in trouble 12 miles off Galley Head during force 12 gale.	Lifeboat stood by until ship got under way
10.06.1956	Motor launch with 6 on Board in difficulties off Garrettstown.	Towed to safety by lifeboat
01.07.1956	French trawler reportedly on fire off Galley Head with mine on board.	Lifeboat searched but trawler reached Kinsale under her own power.
08.07.1956 09.07.1956	Yacht missing in fog off the Old Head of Kinsale.	Lifeboat searched on first day but could not locate. Towed yacht into harbour next day.
24.08.1957	Angling boat in difficulties east of Old Head of Kinsale.	Proceeded to Kinsale under own power.
31.08.1957	Injured man aboard French trawler off Galley Head	Lifeboat could not locate casualty due to incorrect directions.
11.01.1958	Report of a boat having sunk in Clonakilty Bay.	Search carried out false alarm.
23.03.1958	French trawler aground at entrance to Kinsale harbour	Lifeboat recalled as crew were safe.
13.07.1958 **twice.**	Search for missing person at Old Head of Kinsale.	Lifeboat recovered jacket of missing man.

The Sir Arthur Rose Lifeboat (O.N. 801)

23.07.1958	French trawler **Franc Tireur** with injured man aboard 35 miles south of Old Head.	Lifeboat could not locate casualty.
04.08.1958	French trawler **Hoche** of Concarneau aground at entrance to Kinsale harbour	Help from lifeboat not needed but lifeboat returned to stand by while refloating.
02.08.1959	Abandoned dinghy adrift off Old Head.	Search carried out but false alarm.
23.10.1959	French trawler **Hoche** of Concarneau aground at entrance to Kinsale harbour.	Lifeboat went to scene but help not required.
09.10.1960	Motor launch with 2 aboard missing.	Lifeboat returned as Belgian trawler escorted her to safety.
23.10.1961	Report of French trawler in trouble near the Sovereigns.	False alarm lifeboat recalled.

The H.F. Bailey Lifeboat (O.N. 777)
(On Relief Duty)

27.06.1962	Launch **Bluebird** of Courtmacsherry overdue.	Search begun and casualty located.

The Sir Arthur Rose Lifeboat (O.N. 801)

29.09.1962	Motor boat **Puffin** of Cape Clear" aground at entrance to Courtmacsherry harbour.	Lifeboat stood by until casualty refloated.
10.02.1963	French trawler **Fanvette Lozi** taking water 14 miles south each of Kinsale.	Trawler reached Kinsale safely. Lifeboat recalled.
06.03.1963	Fishing vessel **Brigid Caroline** on rocks at Oysterhaven.	Crew assembled but lifeboat assistance not required.

17.03.1963	Man drowned at Dunworley.	Lifeboat carried out search for body.
05.05.1963	Canoe overturned at Garrettstown.	Lifeboat recalled just as she was about to slip moorings.
08.06.1964	Motor launch **Miranda** of Kinsale overdue due to engine failure.	Search carried out and vessel located by Ballycotton Lifeboat.
30.08.1966	Pleasure boat **Sea Rambler** of Cork drifting towards rocks in Dunworley Bay.	Lifeboat towed it to Courtmacsherry.
21.06.1967	Angling boat **Rapparee** of Kinsale broken down south east of Old Head.	Lifeboat joined in search and escorted casualty to Kinsale.
14.07.1967	Pleasure boat overdue out of Oysterhaven with 3 on board.	Lifeboat recalled while on way to search as casualty had turned up.
15.04.1968	Trawler **Rose crest** of Ballinskelligs broken down and drifting near Barrys Point.	Towed to Courtmacsherry by Lifeboat
16.04.1968	Trawler **Rose Crest** of Ballinskelligs developed engine problems again when 2 miles east of Old Head.	Lifeboat towed her to Kinsale.
12.07.1968	Report of lights being flashed off the Seven Heads.	Search carried out but nothing found.
20.07.1968	Fishing launch **Lucky M**e broken down 28 miles south east of Old Head.	Towed to Courtmacsherry by Lifeboat.
27.08.1968	Report of body in water east of the Old Head of Kinsale.	Search carried out but nothing found.

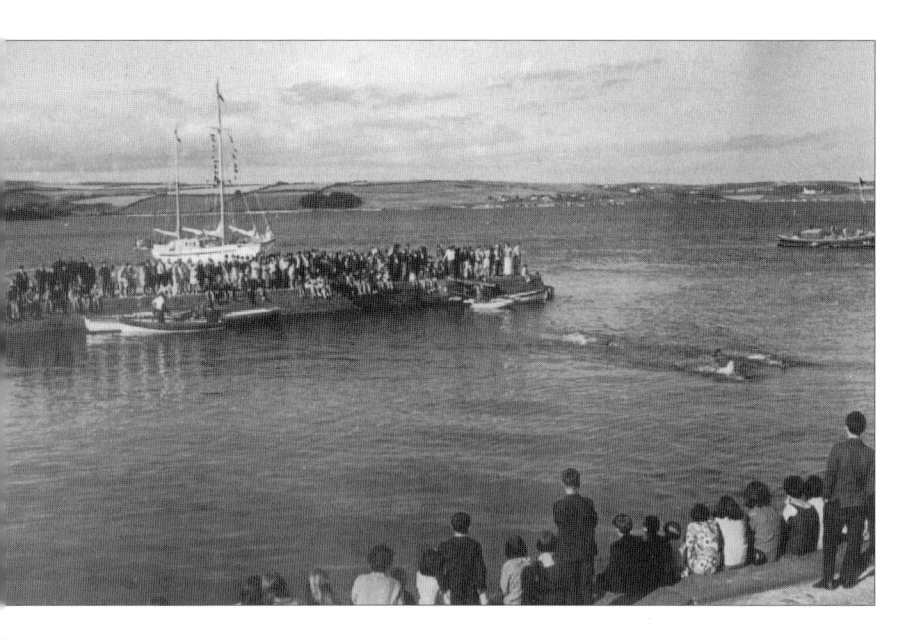

The Regatta in full swing in August 1969, the Courtmacsherry Lifeboat *Sir Arthur Rose* which is soon to be replaced lies at her moorings.
Photograph courtesy of the Cork Examiner.

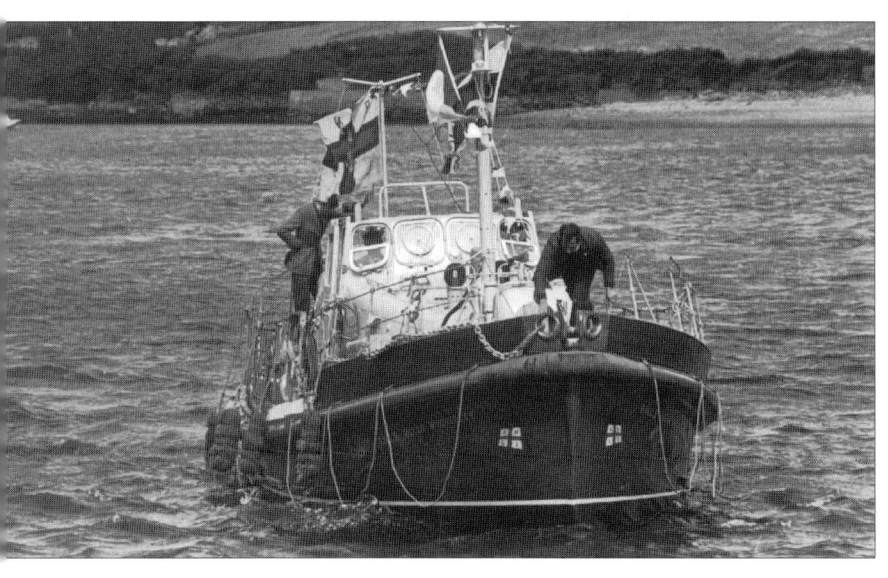

The new Lifeboat for Courtmacsherry arrives at the pier on Saturday August 23rd. 1969. At the wheel of the *Helen Wycherley* is Coxswain John Barry.
Photograph courtesy of the Cork Examiner.

18.02.1969	French trawler **Obeline** drifting onto Old Head of Kinsale during force 10 storm.	Lifeboat stood by all night while another french trawler had casualty in tow.
21.04.1969	Belgian trawler sunk about 40 miles off Galley Head.	Lifeboat recalled as cargo vessel had picked up crew.
06.07.1969	Pleasure launch **Lady Avalon** drifting in Courtmacsherry Bay	Towed to Courtmacsherry by Lifeboat.
15.08.1969	Swimmer drowned at Inchadoney.	Search for body carried out.

The Helen Wycherley Lifeboat (O.N. 959)

14.09.1969	Small launch **Flip** lost in fog 5 miles south west of Seven Heads.	Towed into Courtmacsherry harbour by lifeboat.

The H.F. Bailey Lifeboat (O.N. 777)
(On Relief Duty)

27.09.1969	Sailing dingy capsized at harbour's mouth throwing 3 crew into water.	Lifeboat towed in trawler which had rescued the men.

The Helen Wycherley Lifeboat (O.N. 959)

22.10.1969	Pleasure launch broken down just outside harbour mouth.	Towed to harbour by Lifeboat.
08.04.1970	Lobster boat **Carraig Aonair** broken down near Old Head and trawler **Julia Christian** disabled off Seven Heads.	Lifeboat towed boat to Courtmacsherry Harbour.
21.05.1970	Report of flares at Duneen Strand, Clonakilty Bay.	Search carried out but nothing found.

The Peter and Sarah Blake Lifeboat (O.N. 755)
(On Relief Duty)

14.06.1971	Report of rubber dinghy adrift near Galley Head.	Search carried out but false alarm.

The Helen Wycherley Lifeboat (O.N. 959)

02.07.1971	Two fishing boats out of Ring overdue.	Search begun but Lifeboat recalled as boats had turned up.
26.07.1971	30 Foot motor launch on rocks at Old Head.	Lifeboat went to scene but not required.
14.08.1971	Motor boat with 3 on board capsized east of Old Head	Lifeboat rescued men off the rocks and landed them in Courtmacsherry.
18.08.1971	Motor launch with 3 crew drifting off Old Head.	Towed to Courtmacsherry.
06.07.1972	Trawler **Leo** of Kinsale with crew of 2 broken down South West of Seven Heads.	Lifeboat towed casualty to Courtmacsherry.
26.06.1973	Angling boat **St. Molaga** of Courtmacsherry broken down off Seven Heads.	Towed to Courtmacsherry by Lifeboat.
18.07.1973	16 foot fishing launch with 1 on board missing.	Lifeboat searched from Galley to Old Head but nothing found.
19.07.1973	M.F.V. **Larry O'Rourke** of Courtmacsherry broken down with 5 on board.	Vessel towed to harbour by Lifeboat.
06.08.1973	Report of capsize of rowing boat.	Search carried out but false alarm.

The Michael Stephens Lifeboat (O.N. 838)
(On Relief Duty)

18.03.1974	Person drowned at Owenahincha.	Lifeboat carried out a search.

01.06.1974	Man overboard from yacht **Sybil** in Kinsale Harbour.	Lifeboat searched area.
11.07.1974	**M.F.V. Larry O'Rourke** of Courtmacsherry broken down.	Casualty towed to Courtmacsherry by Lifeboat.
17.07.1974	**M.F.V. Larry O'Rourke** of Courtmacsherry broken down.	Towed to Courtmacsherry.
31.08.1974	Yacht **Cygnet** of Cork on sandbank at Harbour mouth.	Lifeboat recalled.
05.09.1974	Fishing boat **Belrose** broken down with 2 on board.	Boat towed to Courtmacsherry.

The Helen Wycherley Lifeboat (O.N. 959)

25.05.1975	Fishing vessel **Helvic** of Kinsale with crew of 2 broken down.	Towed to Harbour by Lifeboat.
24.08.1975	Fishing vessel **Curliun** of Courtmacsherry disabled.	Towed to Courtmacsherry by Lifeboat.
01.09.1975	Fishing vessel **Curliun** of Courtmacsherry broken down.	Towed to Courtmacsherry.
19.09.1975	Report of fishing vessel in distress	Lifeboat assistance not required.
10.11.1975	Fishing vessel broken down 1/2 mile off Galley Head.	Towed to Harbour by another trawler.
27.06.1976	Cabin cruiser **Repose** of Courtmacsherry broken down in Bay.	Towed to Courtmacsherry by Lifeboat.
08.07.1976	18 foot sailing dinghy sank 1/2 mile off the Old Head of Kinsale.	Lifeboat assistance not required crew got ashore.
02.08.1976	Sailing yacht aground on Old Head of Kinsale.	Yacht towed off by Lifeboat and brought to Courtmacsherry.
15.09.1976	Fishing vessel **Belrose** went on fire and sank in Bay.	Lifeboat went to scene but survivors picked up by other vessel
05.05.1977	Fishing vessel **Naomh Eamon** disabled and taking water 6 miles S.W. of Old Head of Kinsale.	Towed to Harbour by Lifeboat.

The Joseph Hiram Chadwick Lifeboat (O.N. 898)
(On Relief Duty)

19.07.1977	Angling boat **St Anthony** disabled 4 1/2 miles off the Old Head of Kinsale.	Towed to Courtmacsherry.
24.07.1977	Sailing dinghy missing out of Kinsale.	Lifeboat searched and dinghy recovered.
09.08.1977	Report of distress flares off Seven Heads	Search carried out nothing located.
11.08.1977	Fishing vessel **Larry O'Rourke** broken down S.E. of Seven Heads.	Lifeboat towed her to Courtmacsherry.
20.08.1977	Fishing vessel **Moby Dick** with engine failure.	Towed to Harbour by Lifeboat.
08.10.1977	Man drowned off the Old Head of Kinsale.	Body recovered by Lifeboat.

The Helen Wycherley Lifeboat (O.N. 959)

17.06.1978	Trawler **Carraig Aonar** broken down off Seven Heads.	Vessel located and towed to Courtmacsherry.
08.07.1978	Boston Whaler lost propeller near inner Barrels.	Towed to Courtmacsherry by Lifeboat.
20.07.1978	Angling boat **Valhalla** broken down 4 miles off the Old Head of Kinsale.	Lifeboat towed her to Courtmacsherry.
23.07.1978	Small motor boat drifting out to sea near Broadstrand.	Lifeboat towed her to a safe anchorage.
26.07.1978	Bather and Lifeguard in difficulties at Owenahincha.	Lifeboat recalled while on her way to scene.
31.07.1978	Two small dinghies in difficulties near Harbour Mouth.	Lifeboat towed one to Courtmacsherry, other one alright.

03.08.1978	Fishing vessel **Moby Dick** with broken rudder, 2 miles off the 7 Heads.	Towed to Courtmacsherry
06.08.1978	Sailing yacht in difficulties off Garrettstown.	Towed to Courtmacsherry

The Sir Samuel Kelly Lifeboat (O. N.885)
(On Relief Duty.)

07.07.1979	Fishing vessel **Moby Dick** disabled W of the 7 heads.	Lifeboat towed her to Courtmacsherry.
08.07.1979	Two boys adrift in a small dinghy in the harbour.	Lifeboat brought them back to moorings.
15.07.1979	Motor cruiser **Repose** broken down off the Old Head.	Located and towed back to Courtmacsherry.
14.08.1979	Several yachts in difficulties during the Fastnet race including **Casse Tete V**, 26 miles South of the Galley Head.	Lifeboat at sea for 22 hours, towed **Casse Tete V** to Courtmacsherry.

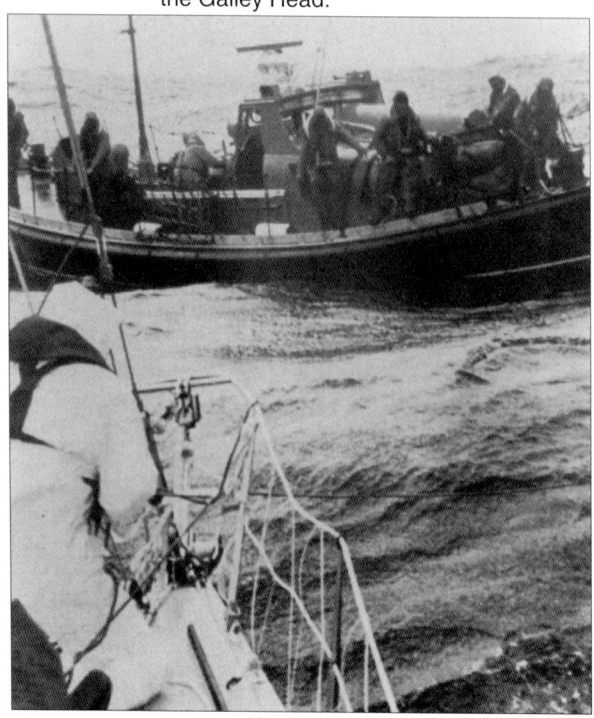

Where did that hill come from !
The tow being attached from *Sir Samuel Kelly* to *Casse Tete V*, off the Galley Head in the afternoon of August 14th. 1979.

Photograph courtesy of Ambrose Greenway.

The Helen Wycherley Lifeboat (O. N. 959)

05.03.1980	Windsurfer missing off Oysterhaven.	Search carried out but casualty had got ashore down the coast.
01.06.1980	Sea angling launch out of fuel near Old Head.	Towed to Courtmacsherry by Lifeboat.
15.06.1980	Angling boat **St. Molaga** lost it's rudder in Courtmacsherry Bay.	Towed her back to Harbour.
30.06.1980	Angling boat **St. Anthony** with gearbox trouble 6 miles South of the 7 heads.	Towed to Courtmacsherry by Lifeboat.
02.08.1980	Angling boat **Larry O' Rourke** broken down S W of the 7 Heads.	Towed to Courtmacsherry.
02.08.1980	Sailing dinghies in difficulty at harbour's mouth.	Escorted them to Pier.
05.09.1980	Fishing boat **Moby Dick** broken down 12 miles South of Barry's Point.	Towed by Lifeboat to Courtmacsherry.

The William Gammon – Manchester and District X X Lifeboat (O. N. 849)
(On Relief Duty.)

23.08.1981	Small boat with a defective outboard motor at the mouth of the harbour.	Towed to Courtmacsherry by Lifeboat.

The Helen Wycherley Lifeboat (O. N. 959)

19.12.1981	Fishing boat **Blue Whale** overwhelmed at Barry's Point in a strong gale.	Search carried out, no trace of owner.
24.04.1982	Motor boat overdue out of Courtmacsherry.	Located by Lifeboat and escorted to Courtmacsherry.
27.06.1982	Speedboat sank outside Clonakilty Harbour.	Man rescued by local boat Lifeboat recalled.

11.07.1982	Yacht **Douchka** of Leamington lost rudder 30 miles off Old Head of Kinsale.	Towed to Courtmacsherry by Lifeboat.
24.09.1982	Yacht **Baxa** of Brittany with gear failure 15 miles south of the Old Head of Kinsale.	Towed to Courtmacsherry by Lifeboat.

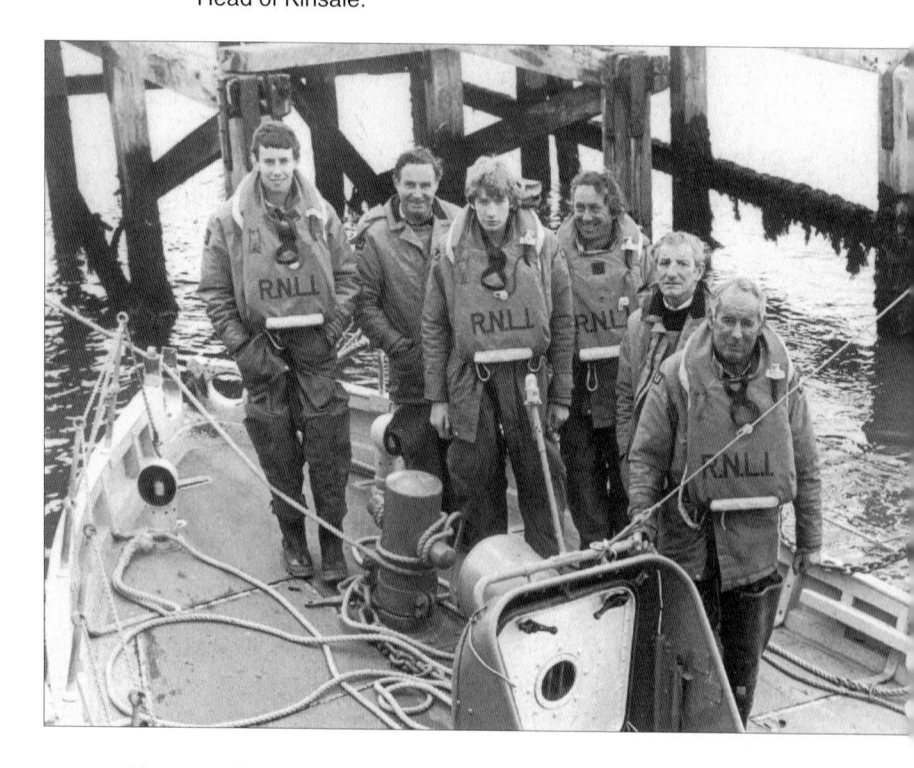

The crew of the Lifeboat after towing in the yacht **Baxa**, on August 24th. 1982 (LtoR) John Madden, Nick Byrne, Colin Bateman, Paddy O'Donovan, Thomas Mulcahy and Brendan Madden.

Photograph courtesy of Michael Miniha

03.11.1982	Fishing boat **Lowland** with fouled propeller at Broadstrand Bay.	Escorted to Courtmacsherry by Lifeboat.
12.05.1983	MFV **Realta Reatha** of Tralee with rudder problems at mouth of Harbour.	Towed to Pier by Lifeboat.

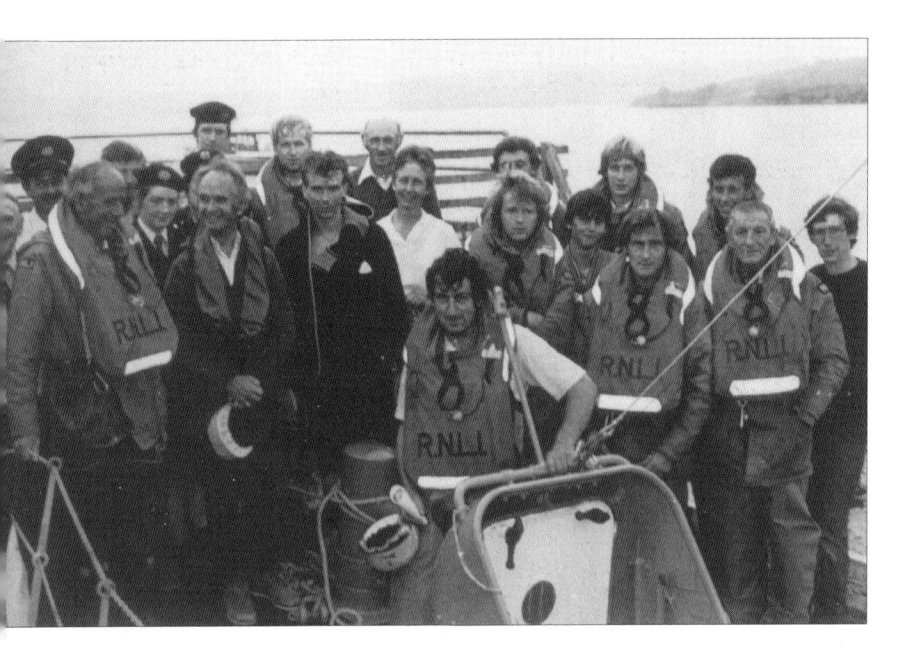

First Aid skills now form an integral part of Lifeboat training and these pictures show a joint exercise taking place with the Irish Red Cross on August the 9th. 1983.

Photographs courtesy of Michael Minihane.

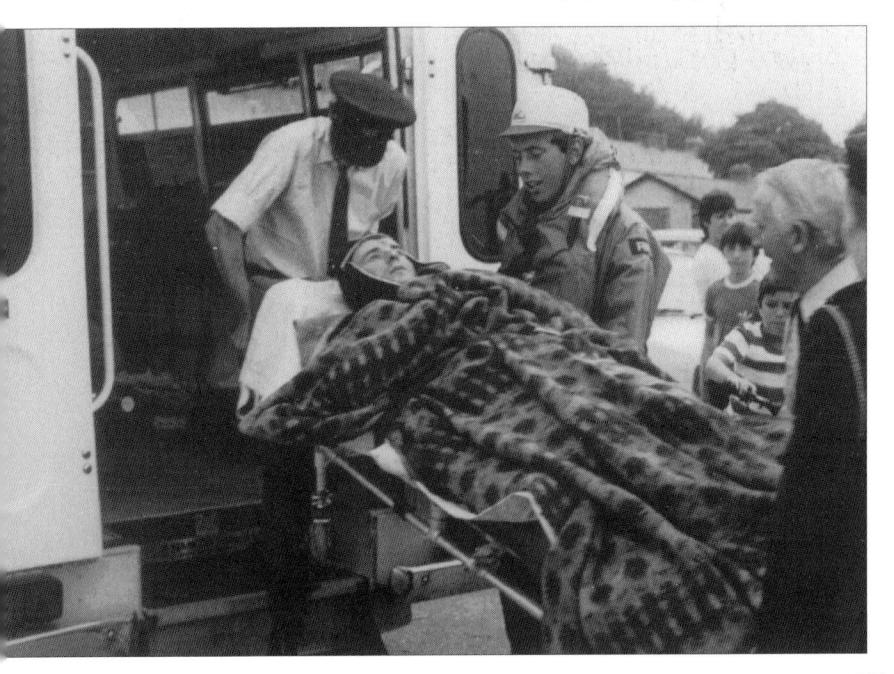

Date	Incident	Action
27.06.1983	Small open boat missing out of Kinsale.	Search carried out and craft escorted to Kinsale.
26.07.1983	Angling boat with engine trouble 10 miles S.W. of Seven Heads.	Lifeboat recalled just as she was about to slip her moorings.
27.07.1983	Sailboard blown out to sea in Clonakilty Bay.	Lifeboat recalled while on her way to scene.
28.04.1984	Man fell down cliff at Old Head of Kinsale.	First Aid rendered and casualty brought to Courtmacsherry on board Lifeboat.
08.05.1984	Motor launch **Irish Mist** sinking near Seven Heads.	Lifeboat crew baled out water as casualty was towed to Courtmacsherry.
05.08.1984	Report of distress flares in Courtmacsherry Bay.	Wide search carried out, nothing found.
08.09.1984	**MFV Lowland** disabled east of Old Head of KInsale.	Towed to Courtmacsherry.
09.10.1984	Man overboard from French trawler.	Lifeboat assisted in search.
21.11.1984	Injured man on board 118,000 Ton ship **Elizabeth** of Liberia.	Lifeboat rendezvoused with ship, S.E. of Seven Heads and transferred man to Ambulance at Courtmacsherry Pier.

The Sir Godfrey Baring Lifeboat (O.N. 887) (On Relief Duty)

Date	Incident	Action
23.02.1985	Sailing dinghy swamped at Coolmain.	Lifeboat went to scene but assistance not required
11.04.1985	Sailboarder in difficulties outside Kinsale harbour.	Lifeboat recalled as another vessel had him on board.
06.05.1985	Lobster boat on the rocks at Barry's Point	Lifeboat stood by as she refloated and escorted her to Courtmacsherry
01.06.1985	Yacht **Feeling Groovy** taking water off the Old Head of Kinsale	Yacht located and escorted to Kinsale.

Date	Incident	Response
03.06.1985	Sailboarder blown out to sea at Dunworley.	Casualty taken on board Lifeboat and brought to Courtmacsherry.
12.06.1985	M F V **Onedin 2** with fouled propeller off Bird's island.	Towed to Courtmacsherry by Lifeboat.
23.06.1985	Air India flight 182 crashed into sea 160 miles S W of Courtmacsherry.	Lifeboat recalled when she was S.W. of Fastnet Rock.

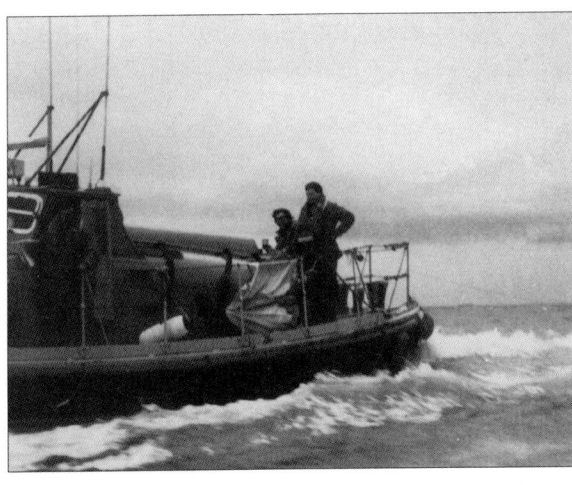

Photograph taken when the Lifeboat was off the Fastnet Rock on June 23rd. 1985. In pre-satellite navigation days the log is streamed from the stern to record the distance covered.

Photograph courtesy of Dermot O' Mahony.

Date	Incident	Response
24.06.1985	Parachute flares sighted west side of Galley Head.	Search carried out, nothing found.
03.07.1985	Lobster boat with gearbox trouble off Barry's Point.	Assisted by another vessel.

The Helen Wycherley Lifeboat (O.N. 959)

Date	Incident	Response
29.07.1985	Fishing vessel Lowland drifting and disabled S.E. of the Old Head of Kinsale.	Located by Lifeboat and towed to Courtmacsherry.
02.08.1985	Sailing yacht **Herself** of Baltimore in difficulties off Seven Heads.	Lifeboat searched but casualty reached Harbour at Courtmacsherry under own power.
08.08.1985	Fishing boat **Beal Boirne** broken down off Seven Heads.	Towed to Courtmacsherry by Lifeboat.

Date	Incident	Outcome
03.09.1985	French fishing vessel **Angoli** aground within Kinsale Harbour.	Lifeboat recalled as crew safe.
03.11.1985	Trawler **Silver Fern** of Dingle broken down 7 miles S.W. of the Old Head of Kinsale.	Vessel located and towed to Courtmacsherry.
30.12.1985	French fishing vessel **Albacore** on rocks at entrance to Kinsale Harbour.	Another trawler assisted, Lifeboat recalled.
31.12.1985	Motor car in the sea west of the Old Head of Kinsale.	Lifeboat stood by.
01.05.1986	Sick man aboard French trawler 28 miles south of Old Head.	Lifeboat launched to provide back up for Sea King.
15.06.1986	Windsurfer in difficulties at Garrettstown Strand.	Lifeboat recalled, man swam ashore.
03.07.1986	Fishing vessel **Jemoline** on rocks under Seven Heads.	Lifeboat fired rocket line to establish tow for another trawler vessel refloated.
13.07.1986	Yacht **Maggio** in difficulties 11 miles S.W. of Courtmacsherry.	Located after extensive search and towed to Courtmacsherry.
03.08.1986	Sailing dinghy in trouble in Courtmacsherry Bay.	Lifeboat recalled as dinghy had got safely ashore.
10.08.1986	Cabin cruiser **Repose** disabled off Seven Heads.	Towed to Courtmacsherry.

The A.M.T. Lifeboat (O.N. 963) (On Relief Duty)

Date	Incident	Outcome
18.09.1986	Small fishing boat overdue out of Travarra.	Search carried out but vessel located and assisted by another fishing boat.

The Helen Wycherley Lifeboat (O.N. 959)

Date	Incident	Outcome
20.05.1987	Small fishing boat drifting onto rocks at East side of Old Head.	Towed to Kinsale Harbour by Lifeboat.
27.06.1987	Fishing boat **Snowdrop** out of Courtmacsherry overdue in thick fog.	Located by Lifeboat and escorted to Harbour.

25.07.1987	Small open boat drifting 20 miles South of the Old Head of Kinsale with 3 on board.	Lifeboat searched all night. Fishermen located by helicopter.

The R. Hope Roberts Lifeboat (O. N. 1011)

15.01.1988	Fishing boat **Darby Greene** broken down in Courtmacsherry Bay.	Towed to Courtmacsherry harbour.
24.01.1988	Boy fell into the sea at Garrettstown.	Search carried out by Lifeboat.
25.01.1988	Continuation of search.	
26.01.1988	Continuation of search.	Lifeboat stood by divers.
07.02.1988	Group of divers in difficulties near Old Head of Kinsale.	Divers taken aboard Lifeboat and their inflatable towed to Courtmacsherry.
20.02.1988	Fishing boat broken down near Black Tom.	Towed to Courtmacsherry.
13.04.1988	Fishing boat **Darby Greene** aground on Horse Rock.	Towed off and taken to Courtmacsherry.
30.05.1988	Small fishing boat with engine problems.	Escorted to harbour by Lifeboat.
06.06.1988	Inflatable dinghy with 8 on board broken down in Courtmacsherry Bay.	Towed to Courtmacsherry.
25.07.1988	Small fishing boat disabled outside the mouth of the harbour.	Towed to Harbour by Lifeboat.
27.07.1988	Two men stranded on a rock at Duneen, Clonakilty Bay.	Rescued by Helicopter, Lifeboat recalled.
16.08.1988	Fishing boat broken down 2 miles East of the Galley Head.	Towed to Courtmacsherry.
12.09.1988	Fishing vessel **Darby Greene** with engine trouble near Old Head of Kinsale.	Towed to Courtmacsherry.

29.10.1988	Windsurfer in difficulties near Garrettstown strand.	Search begun but windsurfer had reached shore.
09.08.1989	Yacht **Shady Lady 3** of Brighton, dismasted S.E. of the Old Head of Kinsale.	Yacht located and towed to Courtmacsherry..

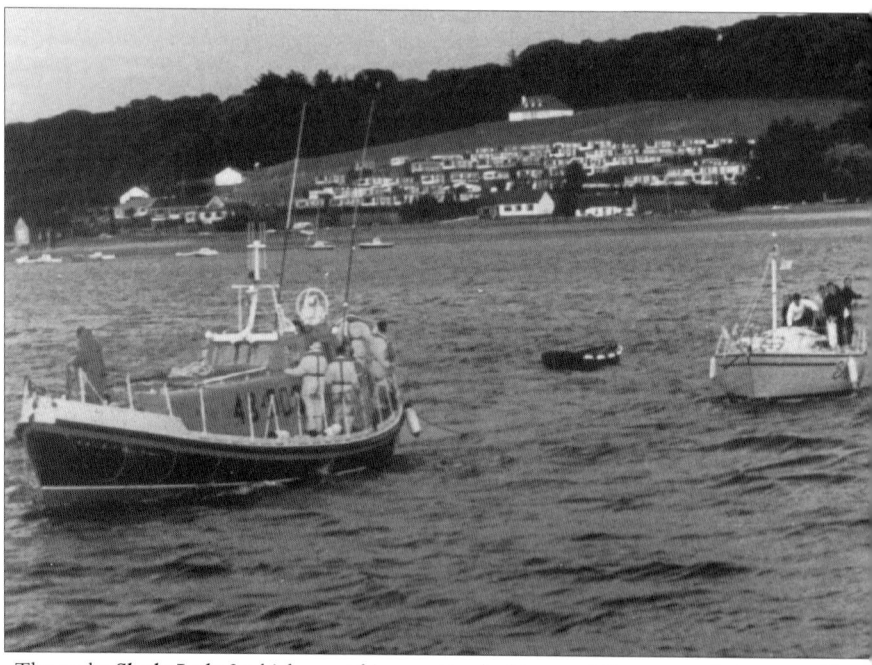

The yacht *Shady Lady 3* which was taking part in the bi-annual Fastnet race, being towed by the *R. Hope Roberts* Lifeboat to Courtmacsherry pier on August the 9th. 1989.

Photograph courtesy of Mrs. Margaret Batem

09.09.1989	Small Trimaran yacht with 1 on board, capsized outside Kinsale Harbour.	Crewman landed in Kinsale and yacht towed in.
09.09.1989	Cabin cruiser **Princess Lisa** with engine trouble east of Kinsale Harbour.	Towed to Kinsale by Lifeboat.
24.09.1989	Alert for small fishing vessel	Crew assembled but alert cancelled.
13.11.1989	Motor boat **Josephine** overdue in fog out of Ring.	Located by Lifeboat and escorted to Courtmacsherry.
05.03.1990	Report of Missing vessel.	Search carried out nothing found.

Date	Event	Outcome
24.03.1990	Fishing vessel **Darby Greene** broken down off the 7 Heads.	Towed to Courtmacsherry.
18.04.1990	Accident on board fishing vessel **Breda Caroline.**	Lifeboat recalled on way to scene.

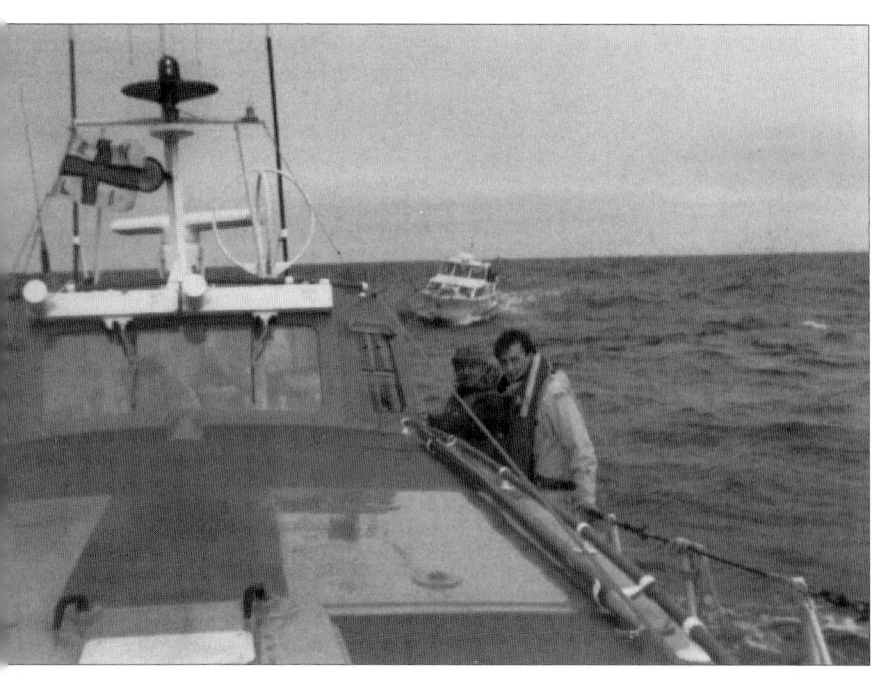

rincess Lisa being towed to Kinsale by Courtmacsherry Lifeboat ***R. Hope Roberts***, on Saturday September the 9th. 1989.
Photograph courtesy of Conor Dullea.

Date	Event	Outcome
20.04.1990	Yachts **Kobold Bleu** and **Turnabout** dragged anchors in harbour.	Lifeboat towed both to pier.
22.04.1990	Youth missing from the Old Head of Kinsale.	Search carried out by Lifeboat, also stood by divers.
23.04.1990	Continuation of search.	Extensive search both out to sea and along shoreline conducted.
29.04.1990	Search for missing youth continues.	
01.05.1990	Cabin cruiser **Ibane Rose** sunk near Dunworley.	Lifeboat recalled as crew had got ashore.

The Jack Shayler and the Lees Lifeboat. (O. N. 1009) (On Relief Duty)

03.06.1990	Two windsurfers in difficulties off Coolmain Point.	Lifeboat took them on board and took them to Courtmacsherry.
26.06.1990	Fishing vessel **Bonaventure** disabled off Galley Head.	Towed to Courtmacsherry by Lifeboat.
29.07.1990	Yacht **Odin** aground at entrance to harbour.	Towed off by Lifeboat and brought to Courtmacsherry pier.
31.07.1990	Report of flares in Courtmacsherry Bay.	Search carried out nothing found.
04.09.1990	Small fishing vessel **(S 164)** with a net around it's propeller off the 7 Heads.	Cut clear and towed to Courtmacsherry.
13.09.1990	Small fishing boat broken down in Courtmacsherry Bay.	Towed to Courtmacsherry Harbour.

The R.Hope Roberts Lifeboat (O.N. 1011)

30.09.1990	Sailboarder in difficulties.	Assisted by Lifeboat.
26.10.1990	Flares reported off the Old Head of Kinsale.	Search carried out in conjunction with Helicopter.
24.03.1991	Fishing vessel **Gaia** of Union Hall broken down 45 miles South of Courtmacsherry.	Located and towed to Courtmacsherry.
16.05.1991	French yacht **Wynduke** of Rouen dismasted 13 miles off the Old Head of Kinsale.	Rigging cut away, yacht towed to Courtmacsherry.
31.05.1991	Fishing vessel **Haul-y-Mor** broken down South of Courtmacsherry.	Towed to Courtmacsherry by Lifeboat.
18.07.1991	Yacht **Iroise** in difficulties near mouth of harbour.	Lifeboat gave help.
23.07.1991	Yacht **Karma** disabled due to machinery failure and small fire,S E of the 7 Heads.	Located and Towed to Courtmacsherry.

Date	Incident	Action
04.08.1991	Yacht **Lullaby** with gear failure in Clonakilty Bay.	Towed to Courtmacsherry by Lifeboat.
08.08.1991	Workboat with engine problems drifting within the harbour.	Lifeboat gave assistance.
04.09.1991	Yacht **Glenduir** on the rocks at East side of the Old Head of Kinsale.	Lifeboat launched to assist but recalled.
15.09.1991	Small open boat with 2 on board overdue out of Kinsale.	Search carried out.
16.09.1991	Searched resumed.	Boat and occupants located by L. E. Orla.
18.02.1992	Report of submarine on fire 14 miles S W of the Galley Head.	Lifeboat launched but alert cancelled.
26.04.1992	Small catamaran drifting ashore at Clonakilty Bay with 2 on board.	Lifeboat rescued yacht's crew.
14.06.1992	Fishing vessel **Coulín** broken down in Courtmacsherry Bay.	Towed to Courtmacsherry by Lifeboat.
22.07.1992	Hoax call.	Lifeboat recalled.
03.08.1992	Catamaran drifting in Kinsale Harbour.	Towed to safety by Lifeboat.
09.08.1992	Fishing vessel Cill Mhuire broken down East of the Old Head of Kinsale	Towed to Courtmacsherry by Lifeboat.
11.08.1992	Rowing boat and occupants reported missing in Courtmacsherry Harbour.	Search carried out but boat located safely ashore.
03.10.1992	**MFV Golden Seeker** with engine problems S E of the 7 Heads.	Towed to Courtmacsherry by Lifeboat.

The Arthur and Blanche Harris Lifeboat. (O.N. 1005)

Date	Incident	Action
06.06.1993	Cabin cruiser taking water in Clonakilty Bay.	Lifeboat pumped out boat until own pumps coped.

25.06.1993	Large fishing vessel sinking 25 miles out.	Alert cancelled.
24.07.1993	Yacht **Dusky Gull** on sand bank at Mouth of Courtmacsherry Harbour.	Lifeboat towed yacht off.
04.08.1993	Vessel reported on fire in Clonakilty Bay.	Lifeboat investigated but false alarm
09.09.1993	Report of vessel in distress.	False alarm alert cancelled
19.09.1993	Report of bather in difficulties.	Alert cancelled.
30.09.1993	Large **M F V Dee Marie** with her propeller fouled 68 miles S W of Courtmacsherry.	Located and towed to Kinsale.
25.12.1993	French fishing vessel **Mustang** in collision with a ship S E of the Old Head of Kinsale.	Lifeboat went to area but vessel had reached Kinsale under her own power.
27.12.1993	Angling boat **Shalimar V** with rudder failure outside Kinsale Harbour.	Towed to Kinsale by Lifeboat.
07.04.1994	Large trawler **Mary Lorraine** on the rocks at the mouth of Kinsale Harbour.	Lifeboat went to scene but assistance not required.

The Faithful Forrester Lifeboat (O.N. 1003)
(On Relief Duty.)

30.06.1994	Man overboard from fishing trawler 30 miles south of Courtmacsherry.	Search co-ordinated by Lifeboat.
03.07.1994	French yacht aground on sandbank at the mouth of Courtmacsherry Harbour.	Towed to safety by Lifeboat.
09.07.1994	Reportof a yacht with rigging failure.	Alert cancelled.

13.07.1994	Flares Reported near the Old Head of Kinsale.	Search carried out, nothing found but yacht assisted at mouth of Kinsale Harbour.
31.07.1994	Swimmer missing inside Courtmacsherry Harbour.	Search Co-ordinated by Lifeboat Body landed at pier.
05.08.1994	Injured angler on board angling boat **Valhalla** off the 7 Heads.	First aid administered, man handed over to ambulance at Courtmacsherry.
09.08.1994	Yacht **Tiger** drifted onto rocks at Blind strand.	Towed off rocks and brought to Courtmacsherry.
24.08.1994	Distress flares reported off the Galley Head	Search carried out nothing found.

The Arthur and Blanche Harris Lifeboat (O.N. 1005)

04.10.1994	Report of a boat in trouble at Broadstrand.	Crew assembled but alert cancelled.
21.10.1994	Alert due to E.P.I.R.B.	Bearing checked using Lifeboat's equipment.
31.10.1994	Two windsurfers in trouble at mouth of Courtmacsherry Harbour.	Both taken on board Lifeboat and landed at Courtmacsherry pier.
01.12.1994	Fishing vessel with World War 2 mine entangled in it's nets heading for Kinsale Harbour.	Lifeboat recalled while underway..
27.01.1995	Alert due to E.P.I.R.B.	Crew on board but alert cancelled.
08.02.1995	Large Ridgid inflatable boat overdue on route from Cornwall to Courtmacsherry.	Search initiated but vessel located.
09.04.1995	Man fell down cliff at the West side of the Old head of Kinsale.	Lifeboat stood by.
28.04.1995	Power boat **Chimes** with engine problems off Garrettstown.	Located and towed to Courtmacsherry.

02.05.1995	Trawler sinking off the Galley Head.	Crew assembled but stood down.
18.05.1995	Report of a small boat in difficulties off the Long Strand.	Crew assembling when alert stood down.
16.06.1995	Sailing craft **Cailín Gleoite** in difficulties East of the 7 Heads.	Located and towed to Courtmacsherry.
09.07.1995	Small cabin cruiser drifted onto rocks near the entrance to Courtmacsherry Harbour.	Towed clear of rocks and brought to Courtmacsherry.

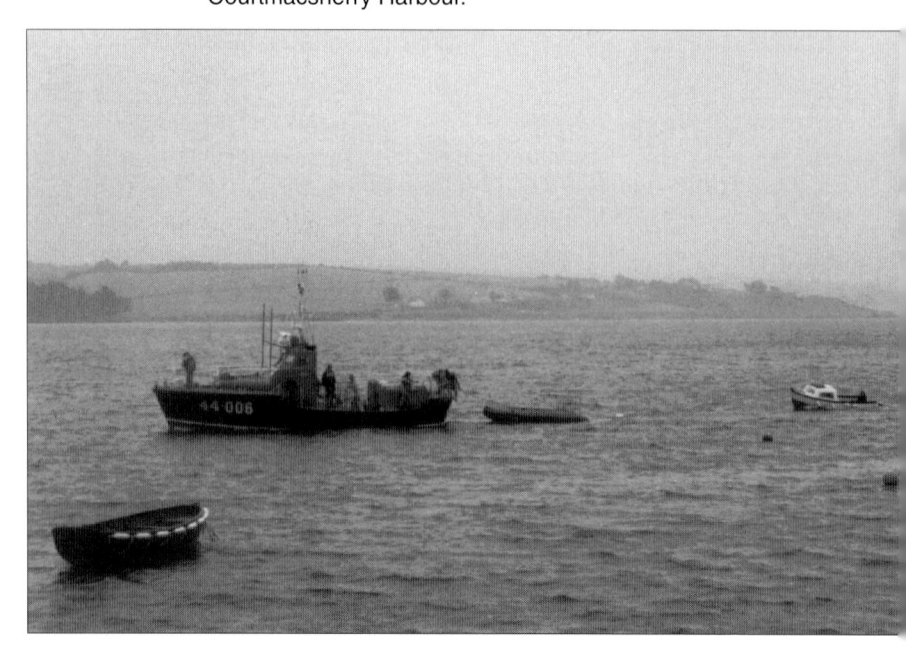

The *Arthur and Blanche Harris* Lifeboat towing the small cabin cruiser to the safety of Courtmacsherry Pier on Sunday July 9th. 1995.(The "rubber duck" immediately behind the Lifeboat, is the author's latest toy.)

Photograph courtesy of Conor Dulle

26.07.1995	Yacht **Aqueous** dragged it's anchors and fouled another moorings in Courtmacsherry Harbour.	Lifeboat took yacht to safe mooring freed anchors.

APPENDIX 2

LIFEBOATS THAT HAVE BEEN STATIONED IN COURTMACSHERRY SINCE 1825

	O.N.	Years
The Plenty	—	1825 – 1829
City Of Dublin	—	1867 – 1885
The Farrant	103	1885 – 1901
Kezia Gwilt	467	1901 – 1929
Sarah Ward & William David Crossweller	716	1929 – 1958
Sir Arthur Rose	801	1958 – 1969
Helen Wycherley	959	1969 – 1987
R. Hope Roberts	1011	1987 – 1993
Arthur & Blanche Harris	1005	1993 – 1995
Frederick Storey Cockburn	1205	1995 –

APPENDIX 3

RELIEF LIFEBOATS THAT HAVE SERVED IN COURTMACSHERRY SINCE THE ARRIVAL OF THE FIRST MOTOR LIFEBOAT IN 1929.

The City of Bradford Lifeboat	(O.N. 680)
The Agnes Cross Lifeboat	(O.N. 663)
The William and Harriot Lifeboat	(O.N. 718)
The H. F. Bailey Lifeboat	(O.N. 777)
The Peter and Sarah Blake Lifeboat	(O.N. 755)
The Michael Stephens Lifeboat	(O.N. 838)
The Joseph Hiram Chadwick Lifeboat	(O.N. 898)
The Sir Samuel Kelly Lifeboat	(O.N. 885)
The William Gammon – Manchester and District XXX Lifeboat	(O.N. 849)
The Sir Godfrey Baring Lifeboat	(O.N. 887)
The A.M.T. Lifeboat	(O.N. 963)
The Royal British Legion Jubilee Lifeboat	(O.N. 1013)
The Jack Shayler and the Lees Lifeboat	(O.N. 1009)
The Faithful Forester Lifeboat	(O.N. 1003)

APPENDIX 4

COXSWAINS OF LIFEBOATS

Noble Ruddock	1875-1901
Tim Keohane	1901-1924
John Moloney	1925
Micheal Keating	1925-1928
Thomas H. Bulpin	1928-1945
Tom Brien	1945-1947
Denis O'Driscoll	1947-1952
John Barry	1952-1974
Paddy Keohane	1974-1977
Sammy Mearns	1977-1981
Brendan Madden	1981-1982
Dermot O'Mahony	1982-

MOTOR MECHANICS

Percy Egan	1929-1946
Denis Daly	1946-1954
Patsy O'Neill	1954-1967
Brendan Madden	1967-1982
Thomas Mulcahy	1982-1988
Mícheál Hurley	1988-

APPENDIX 5

HONORARY SECRETARIES

R.S. Bunbury	1875-1879
Captain H. Townshend	1879-1901
Rev. J.W.B. Forde	1901-1925
Frank Ruddock	1929-1956
Neill C. Mackillop	1957-1962
John Dwyer	1962-1976
Desmond G. Bateman	1976-